The Gift of *Options*

There are other options to help you on your cancer healing journey

By Toni Kimble

A revised edition of The Gift

Sunflower Way Publications
Henry's Life Gifts LLC

Printed in the United States

ISBN- 13: 978-0692322390

ISBN- 10: 0692322396

What Is The Gift of *Options*?

The Gift of *Options* is an essential guide for anyone who has just been diagnosed with cancer and is contemplating a treatment plan.

It offers detailed information of a select and limited group of alternative doctors, clinics, spiritual and nutritional support. We are all very unique physically, mentally and emotionally. There is no one size fits all treatment for everyone. Some of the content can be used in conjunction with conventional medicine. Helpful hints are provided along the way…

Disclaimer

The information contained in The Gift of *Options* is to be used only as a reference to help in the search for complementary and alternative sources of health information. The individuals and/or organizations included in The Gift of *Options* act entirely independently of one another.

The author and creator of The Gift of *Options* is in no way liable for the ideas, theory, practice, treatment or results of any information in The Gift of *Options*.

The author and creator is acting in the capacity of a point of reference only. The beneficiary must use their own judgment and apply the information in accordance with a health care professional.

In The Gift of *Options* you will find many different concepts, theories, research results, ideas, suggestions, and recommendations. The ideas will often sound quite different than other ideas also presented in The Gift of *Options*. The reason for this is that there are many still unfolding avenues for research in the field of both physical and mental health. These avenues originate from quite differing perspectives including food, nutrition, hematology, chemistry, biochemistry, phenomenology, clinical kinesiology, spiritual investigation, and so on.

The creator of The Gift of *Options* takes no responsibility for the degree of past investigation or the level of success experienced by the contributors.

Greatest care was given to provide broad theoretical and practical information set for the beneficiary of The Gift of *Options*.

Thank you.

Toni Kimble

Creator of The Gift of *Options*

Mission Statement

My mission is to enlighten and to help many people on their cancer healing journey. You have options in addition to or in conjunction with conventional medicine, options that not only address the physical, but also address the mind and spirit. I'm planting seeds…

Dedication

I dedicate THE GIFT to our Dad. He will always be one of my favorite people in the world. I admired his simplistic yet imaginative thinking. Dad & Mom were always exploring outside of the box. I am very proud to provide this information in honor of him. It has truly been a labor of love.

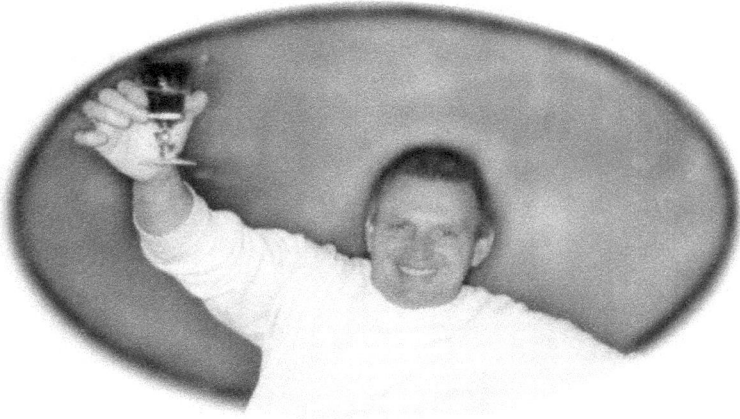

Na Zdrowie !

Table of Contents

Section III

Options addressing the Mind and Spirit

Section IV

Section V

Acknowledgements

Although the idea of The Gift of *Options* was created and executed by me, Toni Kimble, it truly encompasses my family's journey during my Dad's brief illness.

A special thanks to family and friends who have been very supportive, especially my husband Greg, my daughter Savanna (who kept herself busy while mommy put this together) and my immediate family, Mom, Laurie, Paula, and Scott.

This is all for you, Dad!

We love you with all our hearts,

Mom, Laurie, Paula, Toni and Scott

Many Blessings and Hugs,

Toni Kimble

Professional Acknowledgement

With great gratitude I like to thank

Robert Cooney, Esq.

Section I

What is the cause of cancer?

I do not claim to know this answer. However, what is very interesting in researching alternative avenues, many roads lead back to a weakened immune system.

How could your immune system become weekend?

Lifestyle, diet, dental toxins, toxic overload from thoughts and environment could be strong culprits. All these areas may cause acidity in the body which makes it much more favorable for all types of disease to flourish. **Cancer is acidic.** Scientist, Sang Whang, inventor of Alkalife goes into detail about cancer and acidity. Please see the chapter on Sang Whang and Alkalife.

What can you do to strengthen your immune system?

Feed and nurture the body with what it needs physically, emotionally and spiritually!

The human body is miraculous.

The list below is comprised from some of the contributor's information listed in this book and they are only suggestions. Of course you will want to check with your doctor or healthcare practitioner before use.

- Detox program that fits your needs
- Taking specific vitamins and minerals (vitamin D3 is just one of them, but very important)
- Juicing appropriate fruits and vegetables
- Eliminating and adding appropriate foods to your daily diet

- Seek a holistic dentist and evaluate/ fix your mouth and teeth (root canals, amalgam fillings & cavitations)
- Drink clean purified water and drink alkalizing water for therapeutic purposes
- Exercise (walking, Tai Chi, rebounder which is a small trampoline, swim etc…)
- Meditation
- Join a support group (I'm working on putting a network together to connect people who have cancer and can buddy up with them, you are not alone!)
- Get rid of the toxic chemicals in your home
- Laugh- find things that make you giggle!! Shake your sillies out!!
- Find out what you're passionate about and go for it!

Note: **SUGAR!** There is speculation amongst alternative therapies that cancer loves sugar. Whether you choose to believe this or not, most people would agree limiting sugar in your diet may prove to be beneficial.

What Inspired the Birth of The Gift of *Options*?

The Gift of *Options* you now have represents the journey that is near and dear to my family's heart and my heart. You see my Dad passed away of a very advanced case of pancreatic cancer. This wonderful vibrant man fell ill the beginning of July 2007 and passed over in 6 weeks. In such a brief amount of time of my Dad's illness much research and collective information was discovered and continues to be discovered.

Everything included in The Gift of *Options* serves a purpose. My wish for you, the person who has received The Gift of *Options* will have as much information at your fingertips.

Our bodies have an innate intelligence to heal itself if given the right recipe. In my opinion for true healing to take place the mind, body and spirit must be addressed.

You are in charge of your vessel. Your symptoms give clues to help find causes of imbalance. Every one of us is born with special gifts and talents, NO EXCEPTIONS!!

What are yours?! Health and vitality are our natural state of being.

Please take this opportunity to join me to help you on your journey. We are all in this together!

Now, let's get down to business. Since we live in a physical world let's address the physical first. Most people will seek and should seek the advice of an allopathic/conventional doctor. For the most part, they will suggest chemotherapy, radiation or surgery. If you are comfortable with these types of treatments, then by all means follow your heart.

There are other options to help you on your healing journey.

Listed ahead are alternative doctors, clinics, nutritional and spiritual support. They address the body in ways your allopathic/conventional doctor may not suggest or even be aware of. Some of the references included can be used in conjunction with conventional medicine offering a great detox program.

This list provides you with quick informative references. DO YOUR HOMEWORK! Call the numbers provided. Some facilities are located outside of the United States ~ request testimonials. It is best to speak to former patients if you have any reservations traveling and seeking treatment outside of the United States. They will provide you with great insight on your chosen facility. Some testimonials have been included in The Gift of *Options*. It is very important to strictly follow the protocol to receive the most favorable results. The people who "cheated" did not receive optimal results. Trust that inner voice which will lead you on the perfect path.

Let food be your medicine,
let medicine be your food
                    *~**Hippocrates***

Section II

Options addressing the physical Body

Living Foods Institute

The Living Foods Institute, located in Atlanta, Georgia, is an educational Raw and Living Foods Training Center and Therapy Spa. Our center is devoted to teaching people how to incorporate Living Foods into their daily lives with ease and to help people to heal of even the most serious diseases, to prevent health issues from developing and to slow and reverse aging.

Our Atlanta location provides and easy to access state-of-the-art facility featuring a 100% organic hands-on teaching kitchen and therapy spa to help people with nutrition, cleansing and detoxification as well as mental and emotional healing and stress management. The Living Foods Institute was founded in Atlanta and has helped thousands of people from all over the world to heal even when no one thought it possible.

We invite you to come to our amazing Atlanta for the experience of a lifetime.

Brenda Cobb, Founder and Director, overcame breast and cervical cancer without the use of drugs or surgery by following the simple principles of detoxification, optimum nutrition and mental and emotional healing. She also got rid of allergies, acid reflux, indigestion, arthritis, obesity, age or liver spots and gray hair. Her eyesight even improved!

She looks and feels many years younger than her actual age and astounds people with her boundless energy, enthusiasm and charisma. Brenda now devotes her life to educating others in this wonderful Truth.

Learn how Brenda Cobb's Healthy Lifestyle Programs can help you achieve optimum health and happiness through a holistic body, mind and spirit approach to healing.

Hands-on, instructional classes teach you how to get 100% of nutritional value from the foods you prepare while retaining all the enzymes, vitamins, minerals and trace elements you need to live disease-free! Individualized nutritional Programs are designed for each person so they may achieve the health goals and benefits to keep them healthy for a lifetime. There is nothing more empowering than learning to do it yourself and that is exactly what happens when you attend this program. Everyday you are in the kitchen with the best instructors in food preparation. Under their guidance you actually make each of the recipes yourself and learn all of the quick and easy steps to make food preparation simple and fun.

Intensive Programs

The Living Foods Institute offers a variety of intensive Programs including the 30-Day Educator Certification

Program, The 15 Day, 10-Day and 5-Day Programs as well as 1-Day Options to help you begin your detoxification, cleansing and rebuilding process. This Program will empower you to heal your body, mind and spirit and will teach you exciting, new easy-to-prepare recipes that will rebuild your health and give you a new lease on life. You will get increased energy and stamina, glowing skin, healthy hair and nails and an uplifted spirit so you can tackle anything that comes your way with ease, happiness and joy.

Each participant has the opportunity to get in the kitchen and learn by doing. When you complete this Program, you will truly know what to do next and how to put into practice healthy lifestyle principles.

Some of the things You will learn about:

- The difference between Raw foods and Living foods.
- Growing your own sprouts, wheatgrass, sunflower and buckwheat greens and how to sprout a variety of seeds and beans.
- Cleansing and detoxifying your colon, blood, lymphatic system and all your organs and cells

- Exercising, breathing properly and relaxing to manage and reduce stress.
- How to heal the mental thinking and emotional self of issues that may have been buried for years and causing health issues.
- Fasting, over eating, food combining, weight management and healing crises.
- The properties of the most important foods for healing and how to prepare these foods right in your own kitchen.
- The nature of all diseases and the solutions to health problems that plague our society.
- Enzymes, and how these vital elements not only help you heal, but get you in touch with your higher spiritual self.
- Emotional issues and learning how to release the past and old habits and forgive yourself and others so you can go forth with a new enthusiasm for life.
- Organic foods, why they are your best choice and how to become completely sufficient.

You will learn how to prepare Living Foods Meals

In our Programs, you will learn how to prepare a multitude of exciting recipes, so when you get home, you'll know exactly what to do in your home kitchen.

Emotional Healing:

There are emotional reasons behind every illness and just changing the way you eat without getting to the root of the emotional cause is only addressing part of the problem. Feelings of anger store in the liver and many problems with the liver can manifest from chronic complaining, justifying faultfinding to deceive yourself, and feeling bad. Fear stores in the kidneys and kidney stones are actually lumps of undissolved anger. Every disease has an emotional component that is the probable cause. In our Program you will learn all the different emotions that can cause an illness or disease to develop and you'll learn what to do to clear and heal those emotions so the body may heal itself naturally.

Cancer's emotional probable cause is deep hurt, longstanding resentment, a deep secret or grief eating away at the self, carrying hatreds and a feeling of "What's the use?" Diabetes probable cause is a longing for what might have been a great need to control, deep sorrow and no sweetness left. The probable cause of arthritis is feeling unloved, criticism and resentment.

What we think about ourselves becomes the truth for us and every single thought is creating our future. Many of us have foolish ideas about who we are and many rigid rules about how life ought to be lived. Limiting ideas hold us back. When we are very little we learn how to feel about ourselves and live by the reactions of the adults around us. If we lived with people who were very unhappy, frightened, guilty or angry, then we learned a lot of negative things about ourselves and our world. These things accumulate into baggage that we can carry with us throughout our lives.

At the Living Foods Institute we recognize that the most important part of healing is healing the emotions and the spirit and that is why we include emotional healing classes during our programs.

Deep at the center of your being is an infinite well of love. We will help you to allow this love to flow to the surface and fill your heart, mind, consciousness and every cell of your body with its magnificent energy. You will learn to lovingly care for your body, your mind and your spirit. You will learn to live totally in the now and to experience each moment of good knowing that your future is bright, joyous and secure.

In our state-of-the-art therapy spa the very best therapists support each person with specialized therapies to help them heal. Available to our participants are treatments such as Bach Flower Therapy, Body Massage, Chi Machine Treatments, Colonics, Energy Therapy, Q-2 Quantum Footbaths, Indian Head Massage, Infrared Ray Sauna, Medlight Infrared Treatments, Metatron Mat Treatments, Polarity Therapy, Pranic Healing, Rebounder Sessions and Reflexology.

In order to help a person it is important that we know what is actually going on in the body which is the reason we offer the Healthscope Scan which is a most comprehensive test that tells the client their complete physiology including vitamin and mineral levels, heavy metals, food allergies, fungus, mold and candida yeast levels and what is going on with every organ and gland including how the body is aging.

We also offer Thermography, a non-invasive clinical imaging to detect and monitor a number of diseases by showing thermal abnormalities present in the body. Thermography can actually detect tumors in the body up to 8 to 10 years before mammography or other imaging can.

Educational 2-Hour Seminar

For those just wanting to explore and begin learning about Living Foods, we offer a two-hour introductory educational seminar once each month to acquaint you with our Healing Programs, do a Recipe Demonstration, and teach you about the top five things you can do to create optimum health and keep it all your life. There is plenty of time for questions and answers and you will leave feeling empowered and uplifted. There is no charge for this event and donations are suggested which go to our scholarship fund to help others.

You'll learn about:

- The conditions that create all diseases – from cancer to AIDS; heart disease to diabetes – including every minor symptom and every major illness
- The toxic waste dump in your body that could be making you sick and how to clean it up
- Restoring youthfulness and reversing aging
- Transitioning off foods that are destroying your health
- The top reasons people get sick and what to do to heal
- How to take off extra pounds and maintain your ideal weight effortlessly
- The most important things you must do to restore health
- Detoxifying and rebuilding your body at the same time
- The main foods for healing, cleansing and detoxification

- The effects of toxicity and deficiency in the body
- How to live disease free for life
- You'll also get a chance to ask questions about this healthy way of living

Graduation and Banquet Feast Celebration

Once each month we offer the opportunity for the public to come and join us for an incredible organic raw and living foods banquet feast and to celebrate our students' accomplishments. This exciting and extremely motivational event is one of the most inspiring sessions you could ever attend. We do not charge for this event and donations are suggested which go to our scholarship fund to help others.

The Educator Certification Program

The Living Foods Institute Educator Program is for those want to create optimum health for themselves and also learn how to teach and help others in their own communities, cities, states and countries around the world. The Program is 30 days long and is taught in two levels of 15 Days Each.

We have helped thousands of people since opening our doors in 1999 and there are millions of people worldwide who need this type of education and help. The Living

Foods Institute is located in Atlanta, Georgia and is the only one of its kind anywhere in the world. Our mission is to teach this lifestyle throughout the world. God is calling many to help us with this important work. You may be one of these people whose mission is to help others.

Brenda Cobb's vision is to have the Living Foods Institute Program being taught in every state, every city, every country, every corner of the globe, in every language, among every culture, reaching out to everyone around the world in love and peace with a message of hope and healing. If you are ready to become a Strategic Partner and Educator we welcome you with open arms to join us in our mission to "Heal the World One Person At The Time."

Testimonials

Brenda's Story

This is not your typical before and after story. This is the testimony of one woman's all-natural total healing from cancer and how she turned her personal health crisis into a gift for the world.

In 1999 Brenda Cobb was diagnosed with breast and cervical cancer. Her doctor said she would be dead in six months to a year if she didn't do surgery, chemotherapy and radiation. She refused surgery, chemotherapy and radiation. In fact she didn't do anything the doctor recommended and she healed completely by following this Healthy Lifestyle Program!

How did she do it? Brenda nourished her body with organic raw and living foods, detoxified and cleansed her colon, lymphatic system and blood; cleared out and healed emotional stuff she had buried inside and in six months she was completely healed! Brenda used to be plagued with allergies, arthritis, obesity, depression, chronic fatigue, headaches and skin problems, but now that is all in the past. Today she is vibrantly healthy and radiant looking and feeling many years younger than her actual biological age!

Her mission is to teach as many people as possible how to restore and maintain the most optimum health by eating organic raw and living foods, detoxification and emotional healing. She is recognized as a foremost leader, healer and teacher in the raw and living foods movement. Many thousands of people have taken her classes, workshops and seminars and their testimonies are awe-inspiring.

She has authored many books, made numerous television and radio appearances and has taught hundreds of classes about good health and healing naturally. She is a dynamic and charismatic woman who is certain to inspire you to become educated and enlightened and to take care of your most valuable asset, your health!

In 2003 she was awarded an honorary doctorate in therapeutic philosophy from World University and the Phoenix Award from the Mayor of Atlanta for helping the citizens of Georgia to become healthier. Brenda says, "I know that complete healing is possible when a person has real faith and belief and is willing to learn what to do and then do it. There is no disease that cannot be healed! It is imperative people learn how to properly take care of their health. The reason that most people do not do better is because they do not know what to do. This is our main Mission at Living Foods Institute, to educate people how to best take care of their health. When a person becomes educated in exactly what to do, the possibilities are limitless. Everyone can have good health!"

Bridgett Bryant Chattanooga, Tennessee

My adventure to the Living Foods institute is one I never imagined myself taking. At the age of twenty-two I was very much a non-healthy eater, in fact I was a true junk food addict. I had no desire to eat healthy much less learn about taking care of my body. However in the spring of 2007 at 22yrs old I was diagnosed with Non-Hodgkins lymphoma and a rare genetic blood disorder called Hemochromatosis (too much iron in the blood) I was floored and overwhelmed.

By the middle of the summer the cancer had spread. I was extremely sick and under the advice of doctors decided to try chemotherapy. By the second round it was very clear that the procedure was not working. In fact the cancer only began to get worse. On top of that any medicine for the cancer made the blood disorder worse and vice versa. I didn't know what to do. Then towards the end of summer my best friend stumbled upon an article talking about the Living Foods Institute and that Brenda Cobb would be coming to our town to give a seminar. After going and taking in all the information and talking with Brenda, I decided that I would give it a try. My best friend Apryl and I were set to attend the Program in October, however due to my health getting worse I had to prolong it until the Jan class of 2008.

When we arrived I was in the final stages of advanced cancer, I was very sick and weak. The first few days of detoxing were tough. I had so many toxins in my body that were needing to get out but by the fifth day I woke up with energy that I hadn't experienced in over a year. I learned how to take care of my body, why it's important to eat healthy and how to prepare the right food. I was able to work on some emotional issues with Jane and the other wonderful therapies offered from Brenda and her staff. By the end of the Program I felt great and was actually excited about the new healthy life style. I left the center with more energy and clarity and a refreshed sense of life.

Three days after leaving the center I went to the doctor for a full check up to see where the cancer was. After doing the tests over and over the doctors discovered that there was NOT one trace of Cancer or blood disorder in my whole entire body. I am completely healed! I am so thankful that God sent Brenda and her center my way, it was a truly AMAZING experience and most wonderful life style change I have ever experienced.

To read more testimonials please view the website.

Contact Information:

Living Foods Institute

1700 Commerce Dr. NW
Atlanta, GA 30318
Phone: 1-800-844-9876

Email: info@livingfoodsinstitute.com

Website: www.livingfoodsinstitute.com

Individual consultations or group classes are available

Mention **The Gift of** *Options when you enroll a Living Foods Program to receive scholarship help with your tuition.*

Natural Healing Center

Here at the Natural Healing Center we offer a variety of programs. You can experience Dr. Bernard Jensen's Whole Body Cleansing and Detoxification, Dr. Robert Young's pH balance and alkaline nutritional weight loss program, Detoxification program and more. With these programs you can dissolve unwanted weight caused by toxins and you can regain the vitality of your youth and live a healthier lifestyle.

When the pH level in one's body is unbalanced, almost any area of the body can be affected; nervous system (depression), cardiovascular system (heart disease), muscles (fatigue), skin (aging), etc. Even obesity is a sign of over-acidity, a normal body response which protects vital organs from damaging acids and their effects. Conversely, in an alkaline environment, the body reaches an ideal weight and corrects negative health challenges naturally.

Through Live and Dry Blood Cell Analysis you can observe:

- Activity of the immune system
- Parasites, yeast, fungus, mold

- Condition of the red blood cells, liver, kidney, pancreatic, heart, lung, prostate, ovaries, breast and other organ stress
- Features associated with blood sugar imbalance, nutritional deficiency
  crystalline forms, uric acid, cholesterol
- Phenomena associated with gastro-intestinal tract dysfunction and degenerative conditions and more

Viewing of live and dry blood is not a diagnostic procedure for any specific disease. You can see the characteristic of your blood live on a computer screen which can give current information as it pertains to the biological terrain of you (abnormalities appear in the blood sometimes years before they manifest themselves as illness.) This information can assist you by alerting to the advisability of medical referral, or assist you with pH balance and alkaline nutritional detoxification and cleansing program to optimize health and prevent the onset of disease. Health problems may be prevented with early detoxification and cleansing with proper nutritional intervention.

Highlights of the Whole Body Cleansing and pH Miracle Rejuvenating Program

pH Miracle Living Raw Foods with Oriental Nutritional Wisdom

Eco-Friendly Rooms with Spa

Nutritional Live and Dry Blood Cell Analysis

In-Body Composition Analyzer

Gentle Colon Hydrotherapy

Foot Detox Treatments

Far-Infrared Sauna

Steam Room with Herbs

Sunbeam Capsule

Relaxation in Natural Golden Marble Red Clay Room

Hot Tub with Mineral Salt and Herbs

Therapeutic Massage Treatments

MIGUN Jade Thermal Massage

Noble Rex K1 Vibration Exercises

Slant Board Exercises

Deep Breathing and Meditation

Peaceful Beach Walks

Walk on the Beautiful Botanical Garden, 47 acres to the sea

What Does a Whole Body Cleanse Involve?

Whole Body Cleansing

Cleansing the Body From Within

The body heals from within out, from the head down and in reverse order of how the illness began. – Herring's Law of Cure

The secret to vibrant health, youth and vitality is in cleaning the body and mind and then adopting a lifestyle that included clear thoughts, natural foods, pure water, fresh air sunshine and exercise. Learning to cleanse the body and the mind is an essential part of healing. When the body is burdened with toxic waste material, it will be tired and have low immune function. When body is clean, it can absorb the essential nutrients it desperately needs to heal and repair.

Tissue Cleansing Through Bowel Management

Cleansing the body of morbid waste has been done throughout the ages and by people of all walks of life. Those who have practiced tissue cleansing have often saved themselves from severe illness that could not be healed through any other means. Unfortunately, in today's modern society, many know nothing about the healing miracle that can come from cleansing the body.

Dr. Bernard Jensen, Dr. Max Gerson, Victor E. Irons, Dr. Norman Walker, Dr. Herbert Tilden, Dr. Paul Bragg, Dr. John Harvey Kellogg and many others were pioneers in the field of tissue cleansing and have written remarkable case studies in which patients with terminal disease were able to get well by cleansing the colon and the tissues of the body. Dr. Jensen's Tissue Cleansing Through Bowel Management, had guided thousands of people through cleanses and brought remarkable healing results. In addition, Dr. Gerson's book, A Cancer Therapy, presents case study after case study of chronically ill patients who completely regained their health through good nutrition and cleansing.

What Is Tissue Cleansing?

Tissue cleansing involves following a seven- to ten-day program in which one eats whole, natural organic foods (mostly sprouted vegetables) that have been prepared as soft as possible or made into a soup for easy digestion. During the cleanse you will have Alkaline ionized water, herbal teas, broths and raw vegetable juices. In addition, they lie on their backs, in a comfortable position, on a special tissue cleansing system each day. Cleansing the colon allows the body to release old fecal matter that has often been held for years! There have been times parasites of all sort have been evacuated, both living and dead. Those who experience this usually feel tremendous relief, especially if they are, and have been, chronically constipated for years.

Ridding the Bowel of Toxic Waste

Ridding the colon of toxic waste material allows the other organs such as the liver to have a place to release toxins. Cleansing the intestinal villi allows for better absorption of nutrients. Toxins accumulate in the body for various reasons. When we eat three meals a day, colons can become very impacted with old rubbery fecal matter when you do not have bowel movement of time. During a cleanse, this matter, which can look like pieces of an old, black tire, will be very visible. Dr. Rich Anderson, in Cleanse and Purify Thyself, Book Two, calls this old rubbery material "mucoid plaque" and describes it this way:

"Mucoid plaque appears to develop in the presence of acids wherein the mucus is secreted and coagulates. It can then compound with other elements, forming increasingly firm substance. For those who have followed American lifestyle and diet, which is acid producing, it is common for mucoid plaque to form over the glycocalyx, (normal thin layer covering microvilli in the intestines where nutrients are absorbed) of the small intestine, as well as in the small and large intestine. In most cases the layer (or layers) has become intermingled with a variety of damaging toxic constituents. These may include drugs, noxious fecal compounds, heavy metals, pesticides and more depending on what the person eats... Mucoid plaque contributes toward a high percentage of pathological problems, as well as premature death".

Dr. Anderson goes on to say about mucoid plaque that, "This profile weakens intestinal function, causes interference of nerve meridians, and development of bowel disease... Clinical studies have shown that intestinal mucins are frequently altered in such a way as to trigger the evolution of epithelial cells into cancer cells... Gastric carcinomas have also been shown to develop from intestinal metaplasia that has mutated from mucoid plaque".

Where do Toxins Come From?

When people live in polluted cities, or if they smoke, the lungs become laden with tar and soot. Some of this eventually gets carried by the blood into the liver and intestinal tract. Most of the foods and water people ingest today are laden with chemicals, and not all of them are eliminated. Jeffrey Anderson, M.D., and Jerry Stine, in their article "Detoxing From Toxins" stated that: (There are) contaminants that are ingested not by design, but primarily because of contaminated food and water. This category includes food additives, pesticides, agricultural contaminants in meats and dairy products, and heavy metals in fish. Water may contain chemicals and their by-products, pesticides, and heavy metals as well.

Faulty digestion can keep food from being properly processed and sent out of the body. Undigested food remains in the body and creates fermentation, putrefaction and free radicals, which cause us to age way before our time.

In addition, parasites feed on undigested waste material as well as starch and sugar. It is not uncommon for people to have a tapeworm, hookworm, or liver flukes (and these are only a few)! No wonder people are fatigued and can't think clearly. Their bodies are toxic. All of the blood of the body flows through the colon by osmosis and will either pick nutrients that nourish the body or toxins that can cause exhaustion and disease. Cleansing the colon eventually helps to cleanse all tissues of the body and can greatly improve the quality of the blood that circulates throughout the body, including the brain.

So let's wake up from our habitual lifestyles of stuffing our bodies with fast foods filled with processed salt, grease, sugar and chemicals and choose our foods more lovingly and consciously. And let's learn from an age-old truth that one can't put clean water into a dirty vessel tissue!

Cleansing has been used effectively to bring good health for centuries and is still available to those who wish to live healthier, happier lives.

Cleansing Excess Mucus from the Body

There are millions of people in our world today who suffer from excess phlegm in the back of their throats, sinus congestion, sinus infections, stuffy noses, allergies, watery eyes, lung congestion, asthma and bronchitis. Many of our children suffer from runny noses and sinus congestion. More and more children suffer from ear infections and are wearing polyethylene tubes in their ears in order to drain their ears in order to drain the excess fluid from the inner ear through the Eustachian tubes. There are other children and adults who have excess mucus appearing in their stools. They often suffer from constipation, bloating after a meal, digestive disorders, gas and burping. To remedy all of these problems, people are taking decongestants, expectorants, antihistamines, cough suppressants, pain relievers, laxatives, antacids and antibiotics. In the United States alone, 250,000 aspirins are swallowed each day!

Unfortunately, medications treat the symptoms and may suppress the mucus or phlegm for a time, but if the cause is not discovered and treated the problem will persist.

The sad thing is most people haven't a clue as to what is causing the excess mucus production in their bodies. They desperately want it to go away in order not to be so miserable and to be able to get on with their lives. Since the discovery of antibiotics, Americans relinquished the responsibility of their health to "quick fixes" and indeed, antibiotics can save a life. However, antibiotics have been given for everything including the excessive use of antibiotics. There are many antibiotic resistant bacteria today. In addition, antibiotics kill both harmful and beneficial bacteria, such as acidophilus, lactobacillus and bifidus that play a vital role in the work of our immune systems. Other medications have long lists of side effects that people may have to endure as well. It is time we take a long look at how we are living our lives if we want to stay well and healthy. It is time to discover the cause of our problems in order to be able to heal them.

What Is Mucus and What Causes it?

First let us understand what mucus really is and what it does in our bodies. According to *The American Medical Association Encyclopedia of medicine:*

"Mucus is the thick, slimy fluid secreted by mucous membranes. Mucus moistens, lubricates and protects those parts of the body lined by mucous membrane, such as the alimentary and digestive tracts. Mucus prevents stomach acid from damaging the stomach wall and prevents enzymes for digesting the intestines, it eases swallowing and lubricates food as it passes through the alimentary tract, it moistens inhaled air and traps smoke and other foreign particles in the airways (to keep them out of the lungs), and facilitates sexual intercourse.

So mucus in and of itself is helpful and plays an important role in good health. What causes the excess mucus which occurs when people have sinus congestion, lung congestion, phlegm in the back of the throat and mucus in their stools? There are several causes. When the body becomes too acidic, the mucous membranes produce mucus to protect the delicate tissues from the acids.

The body tissues become over-acidic when there is undue stress, lack of sleep, not enough purified water, a lack of fresh air, sunshine and exercise and the consumption of foods that form high levels of acid. As a general rule, everyone is genetically unique and each of us has different requirements based on inheritance, age, position in life and what we have been eating. Most people need to eat more alkalizing-forming foods, which are fresh fruits and vegetables. Processed foods that are high in starch, soda pop, all sweets and alcohol are acid-forming in the body as well. In addition, they have no nutritive value. A large percentage of the American diet is composed of starches, dairy products, meat, salty foods, fried foods, sweets and soda pop. Most packaged foods contain hidden sugars and starches. Americans have consumed so much wheat that many people formed allergies to gluten (the gluey part of wheat). Pasteurized cow's milk contains lots of fillers and no living enzymes to facilitate digestion. Many people have developed allergies to milk or simply cannot digest it. Allergies create inflammation, and allergies to foods produce gas and swelling in the gut causing the body to produce mucus to protect the membranes.

Good health depends upon proper digestion and absorption of nutrients. The small intestine is lined with villi or finger-like projections that increase the surface of absorption area in the small intestine up to a thousand fold. This area of absorption can be dangerously compromised by any condition that irritates the lining of the small intestine. There are also specialized immune cells called immunocytes that line the small intestine. These immunocytes secrete IgA, a crucial component of the mucous lining that makes up our first line of defense. Inflammation destroys these important immune cells, opening the door to intestinal infections, bacteria, viruses, yeast, fungal organisms and parasites.

What to do to Rid the Body of Excess Mucus

If an individual is suffering from excess mucus, phlegm,

sinus congestion, lung congestion, allergies, gas, bloating or mucus in the stool, it would be wise to adopt a more wholesome diet high in vegetables and lower in the acid-forming foods.

Processed foods, foods high in gluten, processed salt, sugar, pasteurized milk products, fried foods, caffeinated drinks, alcohol and sodas should be avoided. Rest, fresh air, sunshine and exercise reduce inflammation and over-acidity in the body and are vital components of good health. Cleansing the colon is also very beneficial.

Three days of our ten day colon and tissue cleanse includes a specific mucus cleanse. This mucus cleanse incorporates alkalinizing foods like sprouted vegetable broths high in potassium as well as herbs that help to expel mucus from the body. We also make sure the intestinal tract is re-inoculated with beneficial bacteria such as acidophilus, lactobacillus and bifidus, and wonderful herbal teas that rid the body of mucus.

To read more detailed information regarding cleansing the kidneys, bladder, liver and gallbladder and what is the "leaky gut syndrome" please visit our website.

Remember, a healthy body does not come from a "quick fix". A chronic illness was never created over-night and it may take a few months or even a year to bring real health back to a sick body. A vibrant, healthy body is earned from the way we eat, drink, think and live!

Our facility offers:

- Dr. Robert O. Young's pH Miracle Living Program
- Dr. Bernard Jensen's Whole Body Cleansing and Rebuilding
- pH Miracle EZ Weight Loss Program
- pH Miracle Living Raw Foods with Oriental Nutritional Wisdom
- Nutritional Live and Dry Blood Cell Analysis
- Colon Hydrotherapy
- Foot Detox
- Far-Infrared Sauna
- Steam Sauna with Herbs
- In Body Composition Analyzer
- Therapeutic Massage
- Jade Thermal Massage
- Oriental Herbs
- Health Products

We invite you to come and meet with Angelo and Chong and experience Jade Thermal Massage System for complementary

Testimony of Kaireen

This is a physical, emotional, and spiritual recovery for me. It's a miracle. I appreciate it <u>so</u> much! I am totally looking forward to changing me.

I was so sick; I thought for sure there was no coming back for me. I had become so depressed. After a lifetime of being abused by doctors and "healers", I absolutely knew not where to turn but inward. I tried everything I knew how to do for myself and what it really came down to was I needed help. More specifically, I needed the right help. The right help for me has been Chong's Natural Healing ten day program and maintenance program.

When I saw the state of my blood, I was motivated. And there was a clear path. A healing path. The changes in my blood before and after the ten day program were so dramatic! It's inspiring! I am really feeling blessed to be experiencing the clarity, energy, and health I feel now. I feel totally renewed, optimistic and about my life and the future and happily committed to staying focused on good health. I give so much thanks to the folks at Natural Healing for helping to make so much possible for me.

Thank you Chong

You saved my life!

Love Kaireen

For more testimonials, please contact the facility.

CAUTION

This program described is not being represented as a cure for any disease or ailment. It is simply a method of cleaning out the bowel and of resorting regular bowel habits, which leads to a cleaner body through more efficient elimination of wastes. The program described here will seldom conflict with any other therapy or treatment, but if you are under a doctor's care, it is best to discuss this program with your doctor and seek his or her counsel and support. If your doctor is interested in natural and preventive health care, he will understand that a clean body is more responsive to any therapeutic measure he feels you need. Our program is not intended to supplant qualified professional health care. Not everyone needs this program, and we are not recommending it as a universal panacea. But, there are many who will benefit from it.

The Natural Healing Center is not a medical facility and we do not give medical advice or treatments.

Contact Information:

Natural Healing Center

Chong Mejias- Director
Coast Inn Spa and Natural Healing Center
18661 North Highway 1
Fort Bragg, Mendocino County, California 95437
Phone: Natural Healing @ 707-964-4914 or
Coast Inn & Spa @707-964-2852 ext. 100
Fax: 707-964-2891
Websites: www.coastnaturalhealingcenter.com
www.coastinnandspa.com &
www.phmiraclehealing.com
Email: coastnaturalhealing@gmail.com

Bio-Medical Center

In 1963 Mildred Nelson founded the Bio Medical Center in Tijuana, Baja California, Mexico. The clinic is located less than 3 miles from the U.S./Mexico border near San Diego California with easy access by air and road transportation from all over the United States and abroad.

Mildred Nelson started work with Harry M. Hoxey in 1946 at Harry's Clinic in Dallas Texas. "We consider cancer a systemic disease, we don't pretend to know its fundamental cause (no one else does either at this writing) but we are convinced that without exception it occurs only in the presence of a profound physiological change in the constituents of body fluids and a consequent chemical imbalance in organism (You Don't Have to Die by Harry M. Hoxsey, 1956, 44-48).

Mildred was the chief nurse and most trusted colleague at the Dallas Clinic working closely with Harry Hoxsey and learning all the protocols. Weakened by a heart condition Harry chose Mildred as his successor and encouraged her to move to Tijuana. "Thanks to Harry the Genius, whose work survives by trusting Mildred Nelson with all our lives" (Peggy Funderburk, Patient-crusader, 1997) Mildred was a teacher and colleague to everyone who knew her. She was a dear friend and remarkable human being.

Over the years Mildred expanded the Bio Medical Center hiring and training a staff of fully licensed, English-speaking MD's. She assembled professional support personnel to see to the care and medical needs of patients who visit Bio Medical Center. Most of the original medical staff and support personnel have remained through the years, and the clinic continues to provide accessible and economical medical help. Before her death, Mildred Nelson took steps to continue her work by appointing her sister Liz Jonas as administrator, "what a remarkable legacy, a legacy that lives on" (Peter Chowka, 1999).

The treatments available at the Bio Medical Center include natural herbs, special diet, vitamins and minerals, lifestyle counseling, positive attitude and conventional medical treatments when indicated. Modern diagnostic methods include extensive laboratory analysis, x-rays, ultrasound, ct scans and other studies as needed on an individual patient. Once an accurate diagnosis has been made, the doctors will outline a special program that works to strengthen the impaired immune system. By rebalancing and normalizing a patient's metabolism, the treatments at the Bio Medical Center give the body a chance to heal itself - often without resorting to more toxic debilitating treatments.

While it should be kept in mind that each patient's illness, prognosis and outcome are different, and that no hospital or clinic can guarantee a 100 percent chance of recovery, there is evidence that many patients – some of them arriving with very late stages of disease – have been helped and their diseases brought under control, by the treatments available at the Bio Medical Center.

Contact Information:

Bio-Medical Center

3170 General Ferreira, Colonia Madero Sur

Tijuana, Baja California Mexico 22046

Bio-Medical Center phone: 011-52-664-684-9011

US #.'s 619-407-7858 and 619-704-8442

Fax: 011-52-664-684-9744

Bio-Medical Email: info@hoxseybiomedical.com

Website: www.hoxseybiomedical.com

The Mission

Of

Health, Healing & Wellness

CANCER - CHRONIC DISEASE - TERMINAL
ILLNESS

The **MISSION** is a Health, Healing and Wellness center
dedicated to Natural Therapies for both healing and disease
prevention.

The **MISSION** is staffed by dedicated healing specialists;
providing Non-Toxic methods now recognized as having
saved the lives of many people who refused to accept the
limitations of chemotherapy and radiation offered to them
in the United States. Just 10 minutes from the U.S. border
patients no longer have to travel to Europe for alternative
treatments

We offer our patients the widest range of non-toxic / no
side-effects natural remedies.

The Integrative Therapy Concept at The Mission is
individually adapted to each patient's particular needs.

The **Mission's** programs are unique because of the range of
treatment modalities available. Our Mission has obtained

therapies from every tradition and developed many more which are available for our clients.

It is now possible to participate in an integrated health program that utilizes the significant advances in the field of Natural Medicine.

Therapies Available

The following is a list of safe natural remedies available to our clients.

- Homeopathic Medicine
- Glyoxal (Koch Vacc.)
- Ridasa
- Cellular RNA Regeneresen
- Ayurveda Medicine
- Immunology
- Fasting
- N-Tumorin
- At Home Treatment Plan
- Mega-Vitamin IV Drip
- Tumor Reduction Therapy
- Auto-Therapy
- HCL Therapy
- Herbal Medicine
- Live Cell Therapy
- Biological Remedies
- Chelation
- Prayer /Visualization

- Color Therapy
- Nutrition &
  Dietary

Frequently Asked Questions

The most important question everyone should ask before deciding on any facility is:

What therapies do you offer and please tell me something about each of them?

Q. What are the fees?

A. Average daily fees range from $400-$600.

Q. Will I receive a home treatment plan once I complete my stay? If so, what does it consist of and how long is it for?

A. Yes, during your stay you are evaluated and assessed for a personalized 6-month at home wellness plan. The plan consists of many different therapy schedules including dietary and nutritional suggestions. This plan is presented to you in consultation prior to your discharge.

This program is unmatched anywhere; no other facility offers such a plan as does The Mission. We invite anyone to show us a similar program.

Q. Will I receive any training and education during my stay?

A. Yes, each person goes home feeling safe knowing that he or she has the knowledge and training to follow the at home wellness plan. Upon arrival, each person is given a multi-page handbook filled with information regarding every phase of their wellness plan. Daily lectures and hands-on training classes for all procedures and life style changes are taught by a staff member.

Testimonial Letters

Maria V.

In February of 2000, I consulted my long time friend and surgeon about the problems I was having with my female organs. He did a battery of tests including ultrasound and found a large Uterine Fibroid tumor and numerous cysts on my ovaries. He recommended I have surgery within 90 days. Fearful of surgery I then decided to consult with the Mission Clinic because they had in the past, successfully treated my son for a condition that I had also been told was hopeless except for surgery. I decided to give their program a trial of 5-6 months. I chose to do the Non-Surgical tumor removal program offered at the clinic. For a period of 6 months, I was to take a group of safe oral remedies by mouth that would have a solvent action upon tumors. With some skepticism, and fearful of the knife I began the program in late February.

During the eighth week of the program, I began to discharge what appeared to be small white flakes. I was scared and contacted the clinic. I was told it was probably the tumor breaking up as this had sometimes happened to other patients undergoing the same treatment. I was passing what appeared to be about a quarter cup daily, this continued for approx. ten days and then stopped.

In May I noticed that my periods were returning to normal. Needless to say I was still scared and thought of having surgery. In June, I contacted the clinic telling them I was considering dropping the program and having surgery. I was told to have another round of tests and ultrasound. I was shocked to see and read the tests. My uterus and ovaries were in a perfect normal state with no sign of the growths and my blood tests were in the healthy range. Elated, I wanted to share the good news with my surgeon. I sat down and presented the tests to him not explaining what I had done. For what seemed like a long time he just stared at the results. Then without asking me anything he threw the test results down upon his desk and stated that this was impossible because the images are clearly seen in the Ultrasound he had taken back in February. He then became angrier telling me to leave his office and that within six months I would be back to see him bleeding to death.

Well, it has been close to three years since I first began having those problems and my periods are normal and I feel I have a new life. The surgeon was wrong when he told me that the knife was the only answer to these growths. Thanks to Dr. Gunier and the Mission Clinic for my healing and continued good health.

Maria V.

May 10, 2006

Dear Mission Center,

Six years ago this past February I came to you with a Fibroid Tumor and multiple Cysts on my ovaries. Well I am happy to report that I just completed my 6 year check-up with my Doctor/Surgeon who originally diagnosed me. He gave me a complete physical exam and ultrasound. He said that I am in perfect health and since the growths had not recurred for the past six years he considers me completely cured. He said that he still does not know what you did for me in Mexico to bring about this miracle but that his hat goes off to you. Well I just want to say I am very grateful to all of you at the Mission and may God continue to bless your great work and heal all the patients that come to you.

Sincerely,

Maria V.

March 2007

Dear Mission Wellness Center,

You performed a miracle on me back in the year 2000 when I came to you with a uterine fibroid tumor and cysts on my ovaries. I recently had my yearly check-up that showed I am in perfect health with no recurrence of my former problems. I had begun treatment with you in February of that year and by June the growths had dissolved away naturally and have never returned in all this time. I am so thankful that I still have all my important organs God gave me at birth and especially thankful I did not have to undergo the awful and expensive surgery suggested to me by the surgeon.

Sincerely,

Maria V.

May 11, 1987

Betty Lee Morales

President

Cancer Control Society

Los Angeles, California 90027

Dear Ms. Morales

I am writing to tell you about a recent treatment experience of mine at La Mission Clinic in Las Playas de Tijuana, Mexico, and to suggest that you include information about this wonderful clinic in your files and mailings.

I arrived at La Mission in March, in a very critical state, cancer in twelve parts of my body including my spine and brain. I was in a wheelchair, medicated for pain with high dosages of Percocet, and unable to eat solid food. Top medical teams at both the Hospital of the University of Pennsylvania and New York Hospital/Cornell Medical

School were finally unable to help me, and my husband and I were in deep despair. The Dr, a kindly, loving physician at La Mission Clinic, agreed to take my case; four weeks later I was sent home relatively pain free, able to eat, with a 24% overall decrease in my cancer levels (obviously, some cancer sites did better than others during this time). I am now on an extended home program and am visibly regaining my health by the day.

The unique feature of his program at La Mission is the fact that it is totally individualized. Extremely sophisticated blood analysis provides a basis for treatment that is geared to the patient's illness in a way that is unmatched by any other program.

The Dr. personally creates a program from among numerous treatment modalities including metabolic therapy, homeopathic medicine, herbal medicine, light therapy, live cell therapy, chelation, HCL and fasting. Each patient's program is different because each patient's body chemistry and illness are different.

Due to the highly individualized nature of the treatment, the doctor and his team only accept a few patients at a time. And devote themselves to patient care like no other physicians and nurses that I have ever seen. The doctor himself personally spent an average of two hours a day with me during my stay, and treated his other patients with the same kind of dedicated intensity.

Before I entered treatment at the clinic I spoke with a large number of former La Mission patients, so I feel confident in telling you that my success is not unique. While I was in residence at the clinic I personally observed other patients experiencing the same astonishing results that I did. I would very much like to share this information with other cancer victims seeking non-toxic alternative therapies. Please feel free to contact me for more information, and to give my name and address to anyone who might be interested.

Sincerely,

Bonnie S
New Paltz,New York

Jan 2007 update: Mrs. Bonnie S. now resides in Florida and is cancer free for many years.

Healing must begin with Love, Patience and Kindness

The Mission, providing care according to Biblical teachings:

To Love Thy Neighbor

and the principals set forth in the Oath of Hippocrates.

First Do No Harm

Love your fellow man as unto yourself, heal the sick, and remove the cause. To succeed, a doctor should be a man endeavoring to follow the footsteps of Jesus Christ, not like the Pharisees in His time, but have the desire to cure our fellow man. Be prepared with unconditional love and compassion to take care of them and above all you must find and remove the *cause* of the disease.

Every sick person deserves three things:

- Quality care.
- A follow-up home treatment plan to continue the good success achieved at the center.
- A loving caring doctor.

Contact Information:

The Mission of Health

Baja California, Mexico

USA Ph. 1-619-662-1578   Mex Ph. 01152-664-631-8283

Mail: 4492 Camino de la Plaza #362

San Ysidro, CA 92173

Website: www.missionmedicalcenter.com

Email: info@missionmedicalcenter.com

Gerson Institute

Healing Your Body with the Gerson Therapy

Throughout our lives our bodies are being filled with a variety of disease and cancer causing pollutants. These toxins reach us through the air we breathe, the food we eat, the medicines we take and the water we drink. As more of these poisons are used every day and cancer rates continue to climb, being able to turn to a proven, natural, detoxifying treatment like the Gerson Therapy is not only reassuring, but necessary.

The Gerson Therapy is a powerful, natural treatment that boosts your body's own immune system to heal cancer, arthritis, heart disease, allergies, and many other degenerative diseases. One aspect of the Gerson Therapy that sets it apart from most other treatment methods is its all-encompassing nature. An abundance of nutrients from thirteen fresh, organic juices are consumed every day, providing your body with a super dose of enzymes, minerals and nutrients. These substances then break down diseased tissue in the body, while enemas aid in eliminating the lifelong buildup of toxins from the liver.

With its whole-body approach to healing, the Gerson Therapy naturally reactivates your body's magnificent ability to heal itself - with no damaging side-effects. Over 200 articles in respected medical literature and thousands of people cured of their "incurable" diseases document the

Gerson Therapy's effectiveness. The Gerson Therapy is one of the few treatments to have a 60 year history of success.

Although its philosophy of cleansing and reactivating the body is simple, the Gerson Therapy is a complex method of treatment requiring significant attention to detail. While many patients have made full recoveries practicing the Gerson Therapy on their own, for best results we encourage starting treatment at a Gerson Institute licensed treatment center.

Please Note: The Gerson Institute does not own, operate, or control any treatment facility. We maintain a licensing program with clinics to ensure that patients are receiving true, 100% Gerson care. Be sure your clinic is Gerson Institute Licensed to provide the Gerson Therapy. Phone the Gerson Institute to discuss how the Gerson Therapy can help you. We will be happy to answer your questions. Within the U.S. call 1-888-4GERSON, outside the U.S. please phone **858-694-0707.**

The Gerson Therapy is a state of the art, contemporary, alternative and natural treatment which utilizes the body's own healing mechanism in the treatment and cure of chronic debilitating illness. When it was introduced to the world by Max Gerson, M.D., the dietary therapy was so far ahead of its time that there were almost no rationales available in the scientific literature to explain how it could produce cures in chronic as well as infectious diseases. But, because it did cure many cases of advanced tuberculosis, heart disease, cancer and numerous lesser conditions, the Gerson Therapy was established as a major contribution to the medical field, through the publication of articles in peer reviewed medical literature http://cancer-research.net/GersonPubs.html. Gerson first published on the topic of cancer in 1945, almost forty years before the adoption of the current official U.S. National Cancer Institute program on diet, nutrition, and cancer.

Max Gerson treated many hundreds of patients and continued to develop and refine his therapy up until his death in 1959, at the age of 78. His most famous patient was Dr. Albert Schweitzer, whom Gerson cured of advanced diabetes when Schweitzer was 75. Schweitzer returned to his African hospital, won the Nobel prize, and worked past age 90. Schweitzer wrote "I see in Dr. Gerson one of the most eminent geniuses in the history of medicine."

Most recently, Dr. Gerson was recognized as a pioneer in his field when he was inducted into the Orthomolecular Medicine Hall of Fame in Ottawa, Canada on May 14, 2005. He joined seven other giants of medicine whose seminal work has been influential in the medical and scientific worlds, and are considered pioneers in their respective fields.

It is rare to find cancer, arthritis, or other degenerative diseases in cultures considered "primitive" by Western civilization. Is it because of diet?

The fact that degenerative diseases appear in these cultures only when modern packaged foods and additives are introduced would certainly support that idea. Max Gerson said "Stay close to nature and its eternal laws will protect you." He considered that degenerative diseases were brought on by toxic, degraded food, water and air.

The Gerson Therapy seeks to regenerate the body to health, supporting each important metabolic requirement by flooding the body with nutrients from almost 20 pounds of organically grown fruits and vegetables daily. Most is used to make fresh raw juice, one glass every hour, 13 times per day. Raw and cooked solid foods are generously consumed. Oxygenation is usually more than doubled, as oxygen deficiency in the blood contributes to many degenerative diseases. The metabolism is also stimulated through the addition of thyroid, potassium and other supplements, and by avoiding heavy animal fats, excess protein, sodium and other toxins.

Degenerative diseases render the body increasingly unable to excrete waste materials adequately, commonly resulting in liver and kidney failure. To prevent this, the Gerson Therapy uses intensive detoxification to eliminate wastes, regenerate the liver, reactivate the immune system and restore the body's essential defenses - enzyme, mineral and hormone systems. With generous, high-quality nutrition, increased oxygen availability, detoxification, and improved metabolism, the cells - and the body - can regenerate, become healthy and prevent future illness.

No treatment works for everyone, every time. Anyone who tells you otherwise is not giving you the facts. We know that when you have been diagnosed with a life-threatening ailment, choosing the best strategy for fighting your illness can be a bewildering task. Everyone claims to have either "the best treatment", "the fastest cure", or "the only therapy that works." In most cases your trusted family physician only has knowledge of conventional treatments, and is either unaware of, or even hostile toward alternative options. No matter how many opinions you receive on how to treat your disease, you are going to make the final decision on what to do, and you must be comfortable with your decision. Choose a treatment that makes the most sense to you.

Most therapies, conventional or alternative treat only the individual symptoms while ignoring what is ultimately causing the disease. The reason the Gerson Therapy is effective with so many different ailments is because it restores the body's incredible ability to heal itself. Rather than treating only the symptoms of a particular disease, the Gerson Therapy treats the cause of the disease itself. Although we feel the Gerson Therapy is the most comprehensive treatment for disease, we don't claim it will cure everything or everyone.

Although the Gerson Institute does not own or operate any medical facilities, we do refer patients to clinics which are fully licensed by the Gerson Institute to provide the Gerson Therapy. Whether you plan to follow the treatment on your own at home, would like to schedule admittance to a clinic, or simply have questions about the Therapy, we encourage you to contact one of our client service representatives at the Gerson Institute.

Caution: Do not start the Gerson Therapy without referring to Charlotte Gerson's book, "Healing the Gerson way" or without the supervision of a Gerson Doctor if any of the following conditions apply:

- Chemotherapy
- Diabetes
- Brain metastases
- Severe kidney damage
- Foreign bodies such as pacemakers, breast implants, steel plates or screws.
- Patients must be able to eat, drink and eliminate normally. The Gerson Therapy cannot be administered to organ transplant recipients.

The Diet

The Gerson diet is naturally high in vitamins, minerals, enzymes, micro-nutrients, extremely low in sodium and fats, and rich in fluids.

The following is a typical daily diet for a Gerson patient on the full therapy regimen:

- Thirteen glasses of fresh, raw carrot/apple and green-leaf juices prepared hourly from fresh, organic fruits and vegetables.
- Three full vegetarian meals, freshly prepared from organically grown fruits, vegetables and whole grains. A typical meal will include salad, cooked vegetables, baked potatoes, vegetable soup and juice.
- Fresh fruit and fresh fruit dessert available at all hours for snacking, in addition to the regular diet.

Medications

All medications used in connection with the Gerson Therapy are classed as biologicals, materials of organic origin that are supplied in therapeutic amounts.

- Potassium compound
- Lugol's solution
- Vitamin B-12
- Thyroid hormone

- Injectable Crude Liver Extract
- Pancreatic Enzymes
- Enemas of coffee and/or chamomile

Detoxification

A very important part of the Gerson Therapy is frequent detoxification of the tissues and blood. This is accomplished through a variety of means, first and foremost through the use of coffee enemas.

The scientific basis for the use of coffee enemas is well documented, and can be obtained from the Gerson Institute.

Patients report that the enemas decrease pain and hasten healing. Biologically, enzyme systems of the gut wall and liver are stimulated, and bile flow is increased. This has been shown to enhance the body's ability to eliminate toxic residues from environmental, chemotherapeutic, and other sources.

Tumor and other diseased tissue is also more rapidly eliminated as it is broken down.

Other means of detoxification include castor oil, used as an additional stimulant of bile flow and as another way to enhance the liver's ability to filter blood. In addition, digestive enzymes serve to enhance absorption of nutrients as well as assist in the elimination of damaged tissue.

Patients must have a complete understanding of the Gerson Therapy so that they may effectively continue the regimen at home after leaving the treatment center. The following are examples of educational opportunities at a typical licensed Gerson facility:

- Gerson-trained physicians and/or educators present lectures and instruction on healing reactions and medication uses.
- Charlotte Gerson and/or other senior Gerson Institute staff members lecture on the theory and practice of the Gerson Therapy, scientific rationales and relevant research.
- Instruction and demonstration of two-piece, press-type juicers, such as the Norwalk Juicer.
- Videotapes of lectures by Charlotte Gerson, other Gerson Institute staff, and Gerson-trained physicians are available for viewing at any time.
- Regular, individualized consultation with your Gerson physician on the specifics of your condition and any necessary modifications to the treatment. During this time, any specific questions you have may be addressed.

For testimonials you can call the Gerson Institute and you will be given names and phone numbers of recovered patients.

Contact Information:

Gerson Institute/Cancer Curing Society

P.O. Box 16138, San Diego, CA 92176
858-694-0707/ 888-443-7766 (US only)
800-838-2256 (US and Canada)
Fax 858-694-0757
Email: info@gerson.org
Website: www.gerson.org

The Alivizatos Treatment Program

A General Overview

The Underlying Philosophy

It is known that poisoning the whole body to kill specific cells has had limited success and generally destroys much of the patient's quality of life. Some patients –actually most patients- will tell you that the side effects from chemotherapy treatments are far worse than the symptoms of the cancer. Surgery has limited success because it frequently doesn't remove all the cancer cells and ultimately becomes a delaying tactic rather than a genuine long-term solution. The Alivizatos® Treatment works on all types of cancer and we will accept patients at all stages as long as they are able to make the trip to the IBC Hospital in Tijuana, Mexico. This treatment utilizes a process that regenerates, enhances and modulates the immune system so that the body can withstand abnormal influences.

Most typical cancer protocols attack other aspects of the patient's health and cause multiple complications, some of which are very serious and debilitating. It is our philosophy to strengthen the body, enhance the immune system and the natural disease-fighting aspects of the patient while starving the cancer and creating a host environment that is not conducive to the growth or reproduction of the cancer cells.

For our program to be successful it is most important for all patients to adhere to what we call The Alivizatos Diet. This diet is primarily low in protein, acids, and dairy products. It is a nourishing, wholesome healthy eating regimen that will be given in writing to all patients at the beginning of their treatment stay. (You can also find that information on the website). The drinking of water is very important to the success of the Alivizatos® Treatment. A minimum of eight glasses of water per day is mandatory to flush the dead cancer cells out of the body.

Who developed this treatment?

Dr. Hariton Alivizatos, M.D., Ph.D. is the inventor/developer of the Alivizatos® Treatment protocol. He was born on the Island of Limnos in the Aegean Sea. While an undergraduate in medical school, he became interested in cancer research and continued four more years of research at the University of Athens, School of Medicine.

Where did it come from?

The Alivizatos Treatment comes from Athens, Greece.

How new is it?

In 1975, with the assistance of his father who had been the doctor in charge of St. Leo's Hospital, Dr. Alivizatos started treating humans.

How does it work?

This treatment utilizes a process that regenerates, enhances and modulates the immune system so that the body can withstand abnormal influences. The treatment pierces the protein and lipid layers of the cancer cells, literally opening the door to the infusion of those cells to effectively begin correction of the patient's metabolism. The resulting effect starves the cancer cells and enhances the condition of the healthy cells. Accordingly, the reproduction of cancer cells is significantly inhibited while the reproduction of the healthy cells is stabilized. The expected result is normally rapid remission and eventual disappearance of the malignancy.

What is in the treatment?

The Alivizatos® serum consists of mega doses of vitamins, minerals and amino acids put together in a complex form. The daily dose is 10cc administered intravenously. Everything found in the Alivizatos® serum is found in the human cell. Inasmuch as the Alivizatos® Treatment is non-toxic, non-biological and non-specific; it is able to pierce the brain-blood barrier, much to the benefit of those suffering from brain tumors. The immune system is enhanced and modulated so that the body can take over control of any disease. If your immune system had been strong, you would not have cancer. It is important to note that this treatment is non-toxic, contrary to the traditional chemotherapy protocols. It is a non-specific enhancement of the entire immune system. Non-biologic means that it is not a vaccine. There have also been significant benefits for those suffering from diabetes, arthritis, emphysema and other related diseases.

How long does it take?

The Alivizatos® Treatment program is typically a 20-day protocol. However, those suffering with Lupus or who have liver involvement are usually prescribed a 30-treatment program, adding an additional 10 to 12 days to their stay.

What about the side effects?

There are essentially no adverse side effects. Patients will most often be somewhat fatigued in the early afternoon during the treatment period and for a month or so after the last treatment. Some patients experience flu-like symptoms during the first week of the treatment period. Hot flashes and chills at times accompany those symptoms but these minor side effects will soon disappear. These reactions are normal and temporary. We recommend that the patient rest as much as possible.

What kind of results should I reasonably expect?

Normally, the patient can expect to see or feel some improvement in the first week but the treatment will be most effective about 30 to 45 days after the last injection and will continue to work for up to six months. As with any treatment, the Alivizatos® Treatment does not help everyone, nor does it claim to do so.

Surgical procedures during the treatment period are not advisable unless an emergency arises. Radiation and x-rays should not be prescribed during or within sixty days after the treatment, as they are deleterious to the Alivizatos® Treatment.

Patients who must receive radiation should consider receiving it a minimum of seven days prior to beginning the Alivizatos® Treatment or wait at least sixty days after receiving the last treatment. If a life-threatening condition should occur and radiation will reduce the size and/or bulk of a tumor, and the patient ops for same, they should consider the administration of booster treatments after the radiation. You must stay alive in order to get well!

What are the current cancer treatments?

There has long been an interest in, and considerable effort expended toward, relieving the pain as well as other acute symptoms and achieving remission of cancer in humans. Presently there are a number of methods and techniques for the treatment of cancer that may include surgery, chemotherapy and radiation therapy. The common characteristics of these techniques, as well as any other presently known technique, is that they are 'Extra-Cellular' in scope. That is, the cancer cell is attacked and attempted to be killed through the application of a killing agent or force outside of the cell. These extra-cellular approaches have been found to be less than satisfactory because of the difficulties penetrating the cancer cell's tough outer membrane. To overcome the protection afforded the cancer cell, in these techniques the attack on the cancer cells must be of such intensity that considerable damage is caused to the normal cells, resulting in severe side effects for the patient. Some of these side effects such as extreme nausea, loss of hair, severe gastric problems, rapid loss of weight and weakening of the immune system, have been found to considerably limit the effectiveness and usefulness of these treatments. At the present time a relatively large number of chemical compounds are recognized for use in clinical therapy for cancer in humans. These anti-tumor agents, most of which have severe toxic effects, are applied by intravenous administration resulting in various therapeutical problems for both the physician and the patient. A safe and effective cancer treatment has been the goal of researchers for a long time. Such a technique, to be successful in the destruction of cancer cells, must be selective in its effect upon the cancer cells, be non-toxic and produce no irreversible damage to the normal cells. In addition, the treatment should reduce the pain normally associated with cancer and restore the appetite of the patient in order to regain normal body strength. We have all had friends or family members who have endured one or more of the above cancer regimes, so it goes without saying that the need to find a safe, non-toxic treatment is as great today as ever before. The Alivizatos® Treatment works on all types of cancer and we will accept patients at all stages so long as they are able to make the trip to the IBC hospital in Tijuana, Mexico. We believe that the Alivizatos® Treatment, although not a "cure," is a treatment that has given quality to and extended the lives of many thousands of our patients. Many have been in total remission for years. This is a safe and effective treatment that you should consider.

What's next?

The Alivizatos® Treatment is only available at the International Bio Care Hospital located about 10 minutes from the international border in Tijuana, Mexico or 35 minutes from downtown San Diego, California where the airport is located. This is a completely modern, full service facility with surgery room, caring, compassionate nurses and is an internationally accredited 27 bed capacity hospital with 7 bilingual medical doctors on staff and other specialists are called in for consultation as needed. Designed with the patients' comfort in mind, there are 15 spacious in-patient hospital rooms. Outpatient facilities are also available.

This program has been administered in Mexico since February of 1984 and the records indicate that some 80% of the patients utilizing this protocol are being assisted as to their quality of life and added longevity. We are able to administer to any number of patients per day since there is rarely any waiting list. We do prefer that patients begin their treatment on Monday due to the availability and scheduling of laboratory facilities. You do not need any inoculations, immunizations, or a visa to enter Mexico. A current passport is mandatory upon returning to the USA.

Why do you need to contact the coordinating office?

To participate in this program, it is required that advance notice be given for both NEW as well as BOOSTER patients.

Please call toll-free 800-262-0212 or go to www.alivizatos.com to make arrangements and to confirm your arrival.

The Coordinating Office of the Alivizatos® Treatment program is located in San Diego, CA and is open office hours Monday to Friday (Pacific Time Zone). All numbers have after hours answering machines and you will receive a callback as soon as possible. The Coordinating Office primarily sends out brochures and can make confirmed reservations for your accommodations on either side of the US/Mexico border or at the hospital. Additionally, the coordinators can answer most of your questions and supply you with the necessary information for your stay while you receive the Alivizatos® Treatment.

The Coordinators will need the following information:
· Name
· Address
· Phone Number, cell phone number, email
· Diagnosis
· Arrival Date
· Who will be traveling with the patient?
· Housing Requirements

The following information is furnished in order for you to calculate the approximate cost of this program.

Transportation:
Costs will vary depending on the distance you travel to get to San Diego, California.

Motels:
Best Western - American Inn & Suites:
Located north of the border in San Diego, California
Cost is approximately $120.00 per day for two people. All rooms have a small refrigerator and wet bar.

IBC Apartments:
Located next door to the hospital in Tijuana, Mexico
Several options are available here starting from $65.00 a night for a one bedroom without kitchenette, $70.00 for one bedroom with kitchenette, $95.00 three bedroom with a full kitchen and $110.00 for a one bedroom VIP Suite. You can get your meals in the dining room of the hospital for $5.00 each meal per person. All prices are in US dollars.

** All prices are subject to change**

What is the cost?

New patients will normally receive 20 treatments after being evaluated with a full medical history and physical examination by the assigned attending physician. This may include a review of past medical record and imaging/laboratory information. These tests will give you and your doctor better information as to your condition and will be done periodically during the treatment period to monitor your progress.

Based on your diagnosis and progress, your attending physician will determine the time and length of follow up or "booster" treatments. You can get an accurate quote of your particular program by contacting us at 1-800-262-0212 or alivinfo@gmail.com

Most private insurance companies in the United States honor claims for medical services from International Bio Care Hospital. We advise you to request more information based on your particular health insurance policy through our insurance coordinating office by contacting us at our toll free number or alivinfo@gmail.com

Payment:
All payments are to be made in advance and in U.S. Currency. We accept all major credit cards. You can also pay by cash or personal check for the full amount at the beginning of the treatment period.

What are the requirements?

At your initial consultation, please provide copies of your full medical records, x-rays, CT Scans, etc. These should include whatever treatment you have had, copies of hospital or doctor's records, (if possible) and your DIAGNOSIS FROM YOUR DOCTOR. Please be sure to get all of your medical records returned to you by your Doctor at IBC Hospital at your last appointment before your homeward departure.

The Alivizatos® Treatment program is being used principally for the treatment of patients with cancer. The hospital will also include patients seeking treatment for emphysema, diabetes, arthritis, lupus and other autoimmune disorders.

What is being offered is not a panacea. The Alivizatos® Treatment protocol does not help everyone and you are not helped overnight. Normally, you will see improvement the first week. As previously mentioned, our records indicate that the treatment will be working for you the hardest some 30 to 45 days after your last injection and will continue to work up to six months.

Contact Information:

The Alivizatos Treatment Program

Teresa Tames, Coordinator
Coordinating Office, San Diego, CA
10050 Vía de la Amistad, Suite 2468
San Diego, CA 92154-7248
Phone: +1 (619) 710-1977 Fax: +1 (619) 414-1404
Toll free 1-800-262-0212

Email: alivinfo@gmail.com

Website: www.alivizatos.com

Testimonials are given upon request

Hallelujah Acres

You Don't Have to Be Sick!

Although it's common, it's not normal to be sick.

God designed our bodies to be healthy. But every day, toxins, free radicals, artificial additives, pesticides and preservatives enter our body from the foods we eat. This depletes healthy cells, which can multiply and become disease.

By following the principles based upon the nutritional plan in Genesis 1:29, you can restore, rebuild, and transform your self-healing body!

Who We Are

Hallelujah Acres is a Christian organization dedicated to helping others discover they can live healthy, vibrant lives free from sickness and disease by simply changing their diet.

It is our mission to help people everywhere experience vibrant health by empowering the self-healing body God created with optimal resources through the principles of the diet and lifestyle described in the book of Genesis.

We have developed a vast library of resources that can help you reclaim your health including free online training programs, hundreds of recipes, the latest health news, live and online events, the world's best health products and more!

Whether online, in person or on the phone, we're here for you!

History of the Hallelujah Diet

Hallelujah Acres was founded in 1992, but the story of how it began dates back to 1976 when Rev. George Malkmus was told he had colon cancer.

In 1976, Rev. Malkmus was a very successful pastor of a large church in upstate New York when he was diagnosed with colon cancer — the same disease that took his mother, despite chemotherapy, radiation treatments and surgery.

Feeling like the "treatment" his mother received was more of a threat than a cure, Rev. Malkmus turned to an evangelist friend, Lester Roloff, who advised him not to go the medical route, but to simply change his diet to raw fruits and vegetables, and to drink lots of fresh carrot juice. He did, and slowly but surely, symptoms began to dissipate and disappear. So he studied everything he could, including the Bible, about this simple way of eating, and found the answers he was looking for in Genesis 1:29.

In 1977, after a year of living this new lifestyle, Rev. Malkmus' baseball-sized tumor had disappeared, as did every other physical problem he was experiencing. His body had been restored!

Sharing The Message of Hope and Healing

This gave Rev. Malkmus a new vision: to tell the world about this change, starting with the Christian community; having been a pastor for 20 years, he felt compelled to share this life-saving information. So, in 1989, Rev. Malkmus wrote his first book, _Why Christians Get Sick_ to share his knowledge and healing experience (today, more than one million copies of this bestseller are in print).

However, most Christians shunned Rev. Malkmus' message. So he began to show that the body of modern medical science supported the wisdom of the original diet given to mankind by God in Genesis 1:29. Those who did listen and who changed their diet, healed themselves. Soon they offered powerful testimonies, making their wellness contagious.

One of these people was Rhonda Jean who, about a year after adopting Rev. Malkmus' message, had lost over 80 pounds, and her arthritis was totally gone. Inspired to share their stories together, Rev. Malkmus and Rhonda were married in 1992.

Recovery Diet Booster

Designed for those with serious health issues, The Recovery Diet Booster option incorporates a more intense version of The Hallelujah Diet to equip the body to perform radical healing in a crisis. The Recovery Diet is in addition to, not in place of the basic Hallelujah Diet.

Why Do I Need This?

Physical problems do not develop overnight — they don't go away overnight, either. But we can help you get on the right track!

The Recovery Diet Booster option gives you the tools you need to begin rebuilding your immune system when facing illness and disease. You'll learn how to address the cause of your illness rather than just the symptoms.

You'll get all the supplies and information you need to fight illness head-on: proper nutrition and digestion, exercise, spiritual nourishment, sunshine, stress management, etc. to empower your immune system to maximum capacity as quickly as possible.

The Hallelujah Recovery Diet

The Hallelujah Recovery Diet is especially encouraged to support your body's healing efforts when battling cancer or other chronic diseases, especially if you are considering or currently undergoing traditional protocols like chemotherapy and radiation.

The concentrated nutrition supports the immune system's efforts at self-healing, often reduces the negative side effects of these toxic treatments, and leads to better results.

HOW IS IT DIFFERENT?

While The Hallelujah Diet provides the body with the resources it needs to maintain great health, The Hallelujah Recovery Diet is intended to increase nutritional power to assist the body in its efforts to fight disease. There are several key differences:

- **Sugar:** The Hallelujah Recovery Diet is very restrictive regarding even healthy sugars because *sugar feeds cancer cells*. Cancer cells absorb many more times as much sugar as normal cells which allows the cancer to grow.
  – The Hallelujah Recovery Diet suggests eliminating all forms of concentrated sugars including refined sugars, dried fruits, fruit juices, honey, maple syrup, and sugar substitutes (except stevia).
  – Small amounts of low-sugar fruit are acceptable. **Fruit intake should not exceed 15% of your total diet.**
  – Vegetable juices should consist of 70% carrot juice and 30% greens to balance the sugar from the carrots.
- **Fats: Cancer also feeds on fats** (and oils) even those considered healthy, like olive oil. Therefore, The Hallelujah Recovery Diet suggests no fats from nuts, seeds, (except flax seed and up to 1/4 of one avocado per day), no oils of any kind except a very limited amount of flax seed oil (men with prostate issues may experience better results when getting their Omega 3 from ground flax seed instead of flax seed oil) and/or **Pharma Finest Pure fish oil** available through Hallelujah Acres.

- **Increased Nutrition:** When fighting disease, it is imperative to remove all toxic foods from the diet (such as sugars and fats) and eat as many raw vegetables as possible. To further boost nutritional concentration, The Hallelujah Recovery Diet DOUBLES the number of daily servings of nutrient-rich **BarleyMax** and vegetable juices (2/3 carrot and 1/3 greens) — one serving every waking hour.

FOR EXAMPLE:

- Start with **BarleyMax** at 7:00 a.m.
- Then a vegetable juice at 8:00 a.m.
- Have another **BarleyMax** at 9:00 a.m.
- Alternate the two juices every hour (skip juice during the lunch and supper hour and extend juices into the early evening).

WHY SO MUCH JUICE?
Juicing is the most efficient way to nourish the body at the cellular level. Alternating the consumption of freshly extracted vegetable juice with a serving of **BarleyMax** on an hourly basis will provide the body with powerful nutrition in an easy to assimilate form. These 12, hourly juices flood the body with a broad spectrum of naturally occurring vitamins, minerals, and trace elements consistently throughout the day, which the body uses to rebuild itself.

ADDITIONAL SUPPLEMENTS

In addition to excellent nutrition and abundant fresh juices, additional supplementation gives the body a concentrated boost of certain nutrients that help the body's self-healing ability. **Hallelujah Acres carries all supplements needed to support this program.**

Toxin Removal: As the body begins cleansing, it is important that the toxins are eliminated timely and efficiently through proper bowel function (2 to 3 well-formed stools daily). A good fiber supplement such as **Hallelujah Acres' <u>Fiber Cleanse</u>** may be helpful to achieve this. (Fiber Cleanse is not designed for long-term use or for pregnant or lactating women. If on medication, consult with your pharmacist for any possible interaction with the herbs in Fiber Cleanse before using.)

Digestive Enzymes: Using 1 capsule of **Hallelujah Acres' <u>Digestive Enzyme</u>** supplement with each juice and 2 to 4 with each meal for the first 3 to 4 weeks will maximize the absorption of nutrients from these foods. Afterwards, reduce to 2 capsules with each meal containing cooked food.

Probiotics: Aggressive use of a good **<u>Probiotic</u>** supplement, such as Hallelujah Acres Professional Strength Probiotic will help rebuild a healthy balance of intestinal flora. The probiotic should be capable of delivering probiotics to the entire digestive tract and contain 10 billion CFU (colony forming units). Suggested serving is 2 such probiotics daily for the first 2 to 4 weeks and then 1 daily thereafter.

Curcumin: Curcumin is the biologically active extract of the turmeric spice, which supplies the body with an abundance of free radical fighting nutrients. Hallelujah Acres suggests one capsule of **Hallelujah Acres' BioCurcumin** daily. BioCurcumin contains BCM-95 which is 5 to 7 times more bio-availability than traditional curcumin supplements.

Iodine: Iodine supplementation supports the thyroid and the immune system. Hallelujah Acres suggests Hallelujah Acres Nascent Iodine Supplementation. It is much more bio-available. Most people - especially those battling chronic diseases - would benefit from a serving of 2 or more vertical drops which supplies 620 mcg of bio-available iodine.

Vitamin D3: **Vitamin D3** offers a broad range of health benefits especially for those fighting serious disease, but sun exposure (especially in winter) is often not enough. Recent research indicates that servings up to 5,000 - 10,000 IU per day may be needed to achieve optimal blood levels. Optimal blood levels of Vitamin D are 50 to 80 ng/ml. Hallelujah Acres offers a superior vitamin D3 supplement (5,000 IU per capsule).

Essential Fatty Acids: When following a plant-based diet, it is important to ensure that a good source of essential fats (omega 3 and omega 6) is available: 1 to 2 Tbsp of flax seed oil or 3 to 4 Tbsp of ground **Flax Seed** daily. If dealing with prostate issues, research suggests the use of ground flax seed rather than the oil. One teaspoon of **Pharmax fish oil** daily will meet the **DHA** needs of the body.

Vitamin B12: This supplement is fundamental to the both The Hallelujah Diet and The Hallelujah Recovery Diet. B12 supplementation is most effective when the Methylcobalamin form of B12 is used in a sublingual form.

After the first 3 to 4 weeks, **Digestive Enzymes** may be reduced to 2 with each meal. **Probiotics** may be reduced to one per day after two to three weeks. **Omega 3** supplementation and other basic supplements should be worked into the schedule as per individual needs. This schedule is not all inclusive and is in ADDITION to the basic Hallelujah Diet - the 85% raw and 15% cooked.

NOTE: We are not medical doctors. We cannot diagnose medical problems nor can we tell anyone how to treat a medical problem. We cannot provide nutritional counseling nor make individual personal recommendations.

Also, consider making an hourly "juicing and supplement" chart so you can visually check off your progress throughout each day. Making a chart helps create a routine that becomes second nature.

PLEASE NOTE: Physical problems do not develop overnight — they don't go away overnight, either. It may take as long as 12 to 18 months of following an aggressive nutrition plan to provide the body with the best opportunity for rebuilding when facing illness and disease.

What's a Lifestyle Center?

It's where you can go for a full immersion experience in living the Hallelujah Lifestyle.

Hearing about the life-saving foods God prescribed for our optimum health is one thing, but it's quite another to live it day by day. The Lifestyle Centers are the fun, comprehensive answer to the often-asked question, "How do you do it—really?"

Each of the Lifestyle Centers is a spacious, comfortable home, and each excels in teaching the preparation and presentation of mouth-watering living foods. Weekend, week-long and two-week packages are essentially the same at each center, but each reflects the personality of its owners and region.

Come by yourself, with your spouse, with friends, or with a

small group for an experience that is often described as eye-opening, joyous and life-changing. You'll get hands-on guidance as you work alongside friends and experienced mentors in the kitchen creating living food recipes. Your expert hosts will show you how to use food processors, juicers, dehydrators, blenders, and other time and labor-saving gadgets.

You'll take part in optional daily group devotions, learn the science and reasoning behind why living foods are healing fuel for your body, and you'll get the daily recreation and exercise your body craves. And at every lunch and dinner hour, you'll celebrate with like-minded friends what you have learned when you eat the marvelous meals you created that day.

Our Goal

We empower you to take control of your health. We do this by providing health-giving knowledge to help you make the transition from the Standard American Diet (SAD) to the Hallelujah Acres lifestyle.

We demonstrate practical ways to live the concept at home, and enable our guest to feel comfortable applying the principles to their everyday lives. In doing so, we offer hope in place of despair, God's peace rather than worldly fear, and concise programs for getting mind, body, and spirit in balance.

By sharing God's desire to see His people walk in divine

health, we are working toward our ultimate goal—to expand the Kingdom of God.

Here's What You'll Learn

- The principles of eating according to Genesis 1:29
- Methods for preparing delicious, healthy living food and juices
- Tips on how to arrange, equip and stock your kitchen
- How to use juicers, blenders, food processors, dehydrators and other time-saving gadgets
- How to live the lifestyle in the "real world"
- How and where to shop for the best healthy ingredients
- How to cut time in the kitchen

As your body adjusts to new freedom from its wearying load of toxins, you'll find new enjoyment in exercise. You'll also discover that your body reacts positively to heath-giving sunlight, so you may find new delight in being outside. And you're sure to make new friends, bonding as you study what the scriptures and science have to say about health, nutrition, and the mind-body connection.

You'll come away from a Lifestyle Center with a restored sense of well-being, revitalized energy, and a renewed spirit.

Testimonial from Plant City, FL

Freedom from Cancer and Fear

I was diagnosed in July 2007 with Colon Cancer – Stage 3 and a 9.5 cancer marker. My tumor was the size of a man's thumb - it had gone through the wall of the colon and I chose to have the tumor surgically removed. Against my wishes, they also removed 32 lymph nodes and we later found out that only one was found to have cancer. The doctor wanted me to start Chemotherapy immediately (just in case) in October 2007 because of that one node.

I did Chemotherapy for three months. By Christmas, I had every side effect you could have from the chemo. Sores in my mouth, chemo-brain, loss of appetite. I didn't want to eat nor did I have the energy to chew. Believe me when I tell you, "Chemo-brain" is something you do not want to experience either. I could not concentrate enough to read and my eyes could not focus on the print and I had no interest in being with friends. I became antisocial which was totally out of character for me. I was filled with fear which had never been a part of my life in the past. There is just something in me that did not want to do anything! I had sleeping problems as well. My life consisted of TV, sleep and doctor appointments The doctor's solution to all the side effects was more and more meds. I'm feeling totally emerged into a deep, deep dark hole that I can't climb out of.

Seeing my condition, a doctor friend of mine mentioned the Hallelujah Acres Lifestyle Center in Plant City – close to my home. But I was so weak from the chemo at this point that I had a hard time making a decision because of all the fear in me. He told me he thought the chemo was killing me which got my attention. I had to stop driving because my reactions were too slow. My family could see how weak I was becoming and put the pressure on me to pray so that I could go to the Plant City Lifestyle Center.

When I arrived in Plant City on January 27, 2008, I was in such a deep hole of depression which made making decisions very hard for me. I booked for a ten day stay and fell in love with the people there. Dave and Sherry were wonderful and I grew to love the new regime I was learning. The first few days I felt were overwhelming mostly because of the chemo-brain but I felt the ten days of juicing and eating right enabled me have the energy I needed to go on.

I believe that my going to Dave & Sherry's Lifestyle Center was surely answered prayer. Upon my arrival, The Orcutt's and my roommate gave me a welcoming hug which gave me a sense of peace and love – I felt the peace of the Lord as I entered their home.

Our Bible Study time was simple but just what I needed and so perfect. Hearing what others had to say and hearing the renewed sense of hope in their voices started to have an impact on me. This all helped to give me the hope that I too could make it. The schedule was excellent and kept me on track. Dave & Sherry pour God's life into everyone and it was evident from the very beginning that all their teaching and the program itself was God inspired. It was at this point that I noticed some of my fears leaving me. The food was amazing – even helped to get my appetite back a little, especially the second week. I fell in love with the relaxation of the hammocks, the morning walks and the fellowship of the other guests. Two months later, I went to my doctor for follow-up blood-work. My liver and kidney function was good and my marker was now a 1.4 (normal is 0-3). I know that this is because of the Hallelujah Lifestyle I am living.

When I arrived in Plant City, I could only shuffle my feet from lack of energy but by the time I left the Orcutt's, I was walking one mile with everyone else. I can drive my car again – and my chemo-brain has improved almost 100%. Towards the end of my stay, I actually slept through one whole night and I am feeling stronger everyday.

I now live with FREEDOM FROM CANCER AND FEAR! I have a whole new way of life and believe the Hallelujah Lifestyle must be taken seriously. All my efforts are well worth it – I have gained a new lease on life. In 2007, I did not know what my 2008 was going to look like, but now this "Little Georgie Girl" is full of life, spunk and I'm Cancer free! Hallelujah!

Georgie Z. – Tarpon Springs, Florida

Please visit our website for more inspirational testimonials.

Website: www.hacres.com

Bring Your Medicines

Hallelujah Acres Lifestyle Centers are not medical supervision facilities. Bring the medicines your health professionals have prescribed. The Lifestyle Center staff does not provide health services such as monitoring vital signs, diagnosing conditions, offering medical advice, prescribing or administering medication.

The Lifestyle Centers are multi-level homes that require the ability to climb and descend stairs.

If you have specific questions about these or other considerations, please contact the center you are interested in visiting for detailed information.

Contact Information:

Lake Lure, North Carolina
Hosts: Tim and Anita Koch
Phone: 877-743-2589
Fax: 828-625-2073

Parkersburg, West Virginia
Hosts: Ben and Janis Medeiros
Phone: 855-556-9341
Fax: 304-489-2976

Plant City, Florida
Hosts: Dave and Sherry Orcutt
Phone: 866-757-1771
Fax: 813-759-2757

Hallelujah Acres Headquarters
916 Cox Road Suite 210, Gastonia, NC 28054
Toll Free: 800-915-9355
Local: 704-481-1700
Fax: 704-481-0345
Website: www.hacres.com

Cancer Free

By Bill Henderson

Hi. My name is Bill Henderson. In November 1990, my late wife, Marjorie, began her **four-year bout** with ovarian cancer. She died on November 1, 1994. Her many operations, chemotherapy treatments and intense pain made her wish often in her last two years for a quick death, or "transition," as she called it.

After watching that, it was hard for me to believe that millions of people each year had to endure that same **torture**. I now believe that the **treatment** she received was the cause of her death, *not the cancer*.

I have read widely in the ensuing years, searching for alternative cancer treatments. I have found over four hundred.

My first book **"Cure Your Cancer"** was the result of my search. First published as an e-book in November, 2000, it quickly became read all over the world, thanks to the power of the Internet. Readers in 86 countries have used the information in that book to become cancer-free. It was also published as a paperback and hard cover book in July 2003. My newer book **"Cancer-Free"** was first published as an e-book and paperback in November, 2004. The newest "Cancer-Free" book is the Fourth Edition, published in November, 2011. It contains all the information I have learned in the seven years since the First Edition was published.

By publishing an Internet newsletter for eleven years to over 34,000 readers, I have built a vast network of cancer doctors, nurses, cancer survivors and cancer crusaders like me. These wonderful people give me daily feedback on what works for them and new discoveries they make.

In fact, one of the holistic physicians who has healed lots of cancer patients has agreed to become the co-author of the latest edition of my book. We are close friends and believe in the same principles about healing cancer. His name is Dr. Carlos M. Garcia, M.D.

You can now listen to my web talk radio show called "How to Live Cancer-Free." Every week, I interview experts and cover new topics related to cancer prevention and healing. Just go to: www.WebTalkRadio.net. There you will be able to listen to my current hour-long show or listen to or download any of my previous shows.

I am not a medical professional, just a **"reporter."** However, I have been able to exchange information among my readers, put them in touch with each other and with doctors, clinics, web sites and other resources. I am proud that I have been able to provide them with much-needed confidence and helped many thousands of them become cancer-free. I will gladly perform the same service for you or your loved one.

My aim with the book, the radio show, the monthly newsletter and the coaching service is to arm you with information. You do not need to be a **victim of the "system,"** as Marjorie was. The power of the Internet will allow you to **co-doctor** intelligently with the knowledge I give you. I will even show you how to find a doctor and dentist who are sympathetic with your quest for a gentle, non-toxic therapy with NO side effects.

My **passion** is to help many more people work around the obstacles of the medical "system" and **conquer their cancer**.

My background is in computer software and marketing. After retiring from the Air Force as a Colonel in 1977, I founded a software company that sold specialized software to architects and engineers. It was the first of its kind in the world. We had clients in 42 states and 4 Canadian provinces. I sold that company in 1995.

In addition to my medical research, I tried several Internet ventures, with some success, from 1998 to 2001. I have a Masters in Business Administration from George Washington University.

My wife and I live in San Antonio, Texas. I have nine great-grandchildren, most of whom live in Michigan. My full-time job now is helping cancer patients like you or your loved one become cancer-free. It is purely a "labor of love."

Cancer Is Easy To Overcome --
I'll Show You How

Join the thousands of people who have read my book and are **free of cancer today** as a result. I've explored the **cause** of their breast cancer, prostate cancer, lung cancer, colon cancer, brain cancer, etc. with them. Together we can **always** determine the cause. Has your cancer doctor discussed the **cause** with you? Why not? Once we've agreed on a cause, reversing the cancer becomes easy. Don't believe me? Please read on.....

Typical causes include root canal teeth or other dental problems (most cancers), emotional trauma and/or long term stress and poor diets.

The thousands who are "cancer-free" include people with all types and stages of cancer, including many *"terminal"* cancer patients. These people are all over the world, in 86 countries. They tend to come to me and my book as a last resort -- after their cancer doctors have given up on them and assigned them a "survival time." "Get your affairs in order -- you have two months to live."

TRASH THAT "DEATH SENTENCE"

I never give up on anyone with cancer. I've seen too many people recover completely after that "survival time" sentence from their doctors. Can you follow a simple diet and supplement regimen for 6-8 weeks? That's all that my readers have found is necessary to reverse their cancer. My mission is to help you join their ranks as a **"long-term cancer survivor."** I want you to live out your normal lifespan, not just "survive" for five years with a destroyed quality of life.

Would you like a method for checking your progress at overcoming the cancer? You prepare the sample at home? You send it to the lab. It costs $55. I give you the instructions in my book.

I'm **not selling anything** except my book and the coaching service I offer (see below). Substances, clinics, doctors, and other resources I recommend pay me nothing. That's how I keep my readers' faith in my integrity. I'm not a medical professional. However, I've studied cancer and its treatment every day for fifteen (15!) years. The information I give you is exactly **"what I would do if I had your cancer."** It's not a prescription. You can "take it or leave it."

BRAND NEW UPDATE

My book "Cancer-Free -- Your Guide to Gentle, Non-toxic Healing" was just updated (4th Edition) in November, 2011. This edition adds Dr. Carlos M. Garcia, M.D. as a co-author with me. Dr. Garcia has contributed lots of his knowledge from his unique experience healing lots of cancer patients at his clinic in Clearwater, Florida. Of course, the book now also includes the information in the 155 newsletters I have published beginning in 2000.

THE HEALING REGIMEN

The regimen I recommend for **ALL** cancer patients comes at the cancer from **seven different "directions."** Seven different theories about how to deal with cancer cells. All of these seven forms of treatment are **gentle** (no dangerous, too-rapid "die off"), **non-toxic** and they all work together. They are, in fact, synergistic. They help each other.

They address the five characteristics of every cancer. These five conditions **must be corrected before anyone can get over cancer:** 1) A weak immune system; 2) A lack of oxygen uptake by the cells; 3) Excessive toxins; 4) Acidity; and 5) Specific deficiencies. Conventional cancer treatment (chemotherapy, radiation and surgery) makes all of these conditions worse. In fact, it is responsible for almost all the deaths attributed to "cancer." That's right. The "treatment" causes the deaths -- not the cancer.

Why? The conventional cancer treatments are approaching the cancer tumor (or its existence in your blood, lymph system or bone marrow) as if it were the "enemy." Kill the cancer cells at all costs! Those costs may be your heart, your liver, your kidneys -- or your life.

Why do they do these things? There are literally 400 other effective ways to treat cancer. All of them are non-toxic and harmless to your other organs. Why doesn't your cancer doctor tell you about these options?

Can you spell **M-O-N-E-Y?**

The average cancer patient (like you) generates $1.3 million in revenue for the cancer "industry." Do you think they want you to be healed by something that costs pennies a day?

THE COST

How much would you think a regimen like mine should cost? Take a guess. $10,000 US Dollars? $2,500 US Dollars a month? Well, hold onto your chair. The cost is exactly **$155 per month** in U.S. Dollars. Please understand. You pay just $155 for the food and supplements. **You don't pay me anything.** I don't get any compensation from the sources where I recommend you buy the food and supplements. I just try to give you the cheapest and best source I can find. I have often changed my recommendations when I have found something better.

MY CRUSADE

To get to this regimen, I have studied cancer treatment every day for the last **fifteen years** -- since 1998, when I first realized all the information that was available even then on the Internet. I've sifted through hundreds of "alternative" cancer "cures." I've talked to thousands of cancer survivors, cancer doctors, nutritionists, nurses, cancer experts of all kinds. I've read everything I could get my hands on. I am on a mission -- **a crusade**, if you will -- to help as many people as possible avoid my late wife's fate. [See "About Me" on the left of this screen.]

JUST A LIMITED TIME COMMITMENT

Now, you or your loved one can benefit from my experience. All I suggest is that you give this regimen six to eight weeks while postponing other treatment. I'm not asking for you to commit your life -- just six to eight weeks. I've found that within just a few days, 90% or more of the cancer patients who do this feel so much better that they continue with this regimen **for life**.

You see, I know it's not too difficult because I do it every day myself **for prevention.** I am 82 years old and in perfect health.

ADDITIONAL COACHING

To overcome cancer, it is important to have your loved ones "on board" with you. To make it easy to do that, just explore the Coaching service I offer at this website. The information in this Coaching service comes from the lessons I've learned from all my research, but, more importantly, from the lessons taught to me by all the thousands of coaching clients I've worked with all over the world. It is in a format now where you can easily share it with your loved ones.

A SIMPLE APPROACH

How does this work? Simple.

First, you buy my book, either in e-book (computer file) form or in paperback form. Included in the book is a complete set of instructions on the "Self-Treatments That I Recommend." There is also information on locating holistic doctors, clinics and other resources. Usually you do not need a holistic doctor or clinic.

Second, you test the levels of cancer cells in your body using a test I teach you about in the book.

Third, you try my recommended regimen for 6-8 weeks.

Fourth, you take a second test. If that test shows you are not making progress (rare for people who have the discipline to follow my recommendations), you come back to this website and click on the "Coaching" link. Just follow the instructions there to get **coaching from me** anywhere in the world. We will discuss the causes of your cancer, how to reverse them, and then what to try next, based on your experience to that point.

Deal?

I'm committed to helping you. If you can commit to just this six to eight week program at a cost of **less than $200,** including the price of my book, the special food and the supplements, we have a deal.

Interested? Remember: The first step to complete and permanent healing is to buy my book "Cancer-Free."

FREE NEWSLETTER

You may also want to subscribe to my free "Cancer-Free" newsletter. I publish it by e-mail every month. It updates the information in the book with anything new I've discovered. Usually, I publish the story of a successful cancer survivor. The sign-up routine is on almost every page of my website (see below).

Bill Henderson
Author, "Cure Your Cancer" and "Cancer-Free"

<u>Alternative Cancer Treatment Information</u>
Here are some stories from cancer patients and others about their healing experience. Just click on the link above.

Coaching For You

READY FOR SOME PERSONAL COACHING?

OK, now that you've read Dr. Garcia's and my book, Cancer-Free (4th Edition), you may want to talk to someone who knows what causes cancer and how to get over it. That's me. I've been learning that from my experience working with the thousands of wonderful people who I've helped heal their cancers in the last 16 years.

<u>Here's a testimonial about my coaching service:</u>

I would like to express my gratitude for the work you do. For those of us facing cancer and wanting to do it alternatively it can be a very difficult road with many unclear paths. Your work makes this journey so much clearer and provides hope...you have restored hope, and I believe hope is what it takes to truly heal. Thank you for your support. I send you back all the blessings you have given me. I have no doubt your work will continue to heal and bring peace to many.

Take care, Camey Martinez

Thank you, Camey. That's what I hear all the time......hope! If there is anything you cannot get from the cancer doctors, it is hope. All they seem to be able to dish out are "death sentences." Well, you have come to the right place if you want hope. I've seen so many "miracles," I never give up on anyone.

COACHING SERVICE OVERVIEW

I've provided this service for people in 64 countries. Their problems are the same. They all need the specific information I can give them about "what I would do if it were me." They all want to share it with their loved ones who are helping them.

There is very valuable information available to you as soon as you sign up for this coaching service. You get a personalized and **easy to use** "portal." You simply enter your email address and password to do the following:

* Schedule a phone or Skype online video conference where we get acquainted
* Securely and easily email me as often as you like to get my guidance and suggestions
* Watch educational videos from me on different topics to view at your convenience
* Read pertinent articles, including a list of dentists and doctors I trust, to share with your loved ones
* Access to some of the better Web Talk Radio interviews I've done

* Continued, unlimited access to me for six months after you sign up

SHARING COACHING INFORMATION WITH LOVED ONES -- VITAL!

Anytime you like, and as often as you like, you can share your videos and other information with your loved ones. It's easy. They want to help you, so they need the information you have and they need to understand why you are doing what you're doing. It really helps to share the videos, articles, or any of your information with your family and friends. Maybe they want to listen in on the call we do. That's fine too!

Here are more testimonials from grateful "coachees."

Bill, please allow my voice to join thousands of others worldwide to thank you from the deepest part of my soul for what you are doing for us and our loved ones. Your kindness and compassion shine through in each word, and you are an inspiration to all of us.

- Sending hugs, Anne Loeser

I want to say that my admiration, respect, and appreciation for the work you do are all immense. Your gift to humanity is truly extraordinary, and you have brought so much help and confidence to my family just by your sharing the extremely valuable information you have provided to us in your books, your coaching and your many podcasts. You are truly a hero for me and my family and friends. Thanks from the bottom of my heart for being you, Bill.

- Sincerely, Jim Duffy

Good day to you and thank you once again for all your precious information. We found it very informative and useful to help our loved ones, family members and friends.

We highly appreciate your kind assistance and we shall give you more feedback on my father-in-law's health after his change in diet. Thank you once again.

- Warm regards, Cathy Wong

I can't thank you enough for all the work you have done. I have been researching alternative cancer therapies for 15 years since losing both of my parents to this terrible disease. I can say without question you have put together the most complete, simple yet comprehensive resource that I have yet found. Most important it is practical and useable information that will make a difference for anyone willing to implement the program and stick with it.

- Best regards, Charles Froeming

So, ready to sign up? The cost for my easy to follow coaching service is just a one-time payment of $195 for six months of contact with me (just $1.06 a day). I look forward to helping you.   Just go to my website (see below) and click on the Coaching page.

Bill Henderson
Author and Cancer Coach

Contact Information:

Bill Henderson

Website: www.beating-cancer-gently.com

Email: uhealcancer@gmail.com

Denise Abda, MT(ASCP),IMA,HC(AADP)

www.findyourfountain.com

Regaining your health through education, knowledge and awareness.

Health, Nutrition and Wellness

Denise Abda's introduction to holistic health and wellness began after she exhausted traditional therapies for her own health problems. Through research into nutrition and understanding the awareness of acid/alkaline balance for the body, she teaches the importance of food choices and how it affects your health.

Ms Abda is a graduate of the University of Scranton with a BS in Biochemistry. Prior to becoming a health consultant, she was employed at Community Medical Center in Scranton, Pennsylvania as a Medical Technologist (MT), certified by the American Society of Clinical Pathology. She furthered her education by studying under microbiologist, Robert O. Young, MS,DSc,PhD,ND at the pH Miracle Center in San Diego, CA, earning her certification in Microscopy (IMA) in 2003. She has also graduated from The Institute of Integrative Nutrition in NYC where she earned certification from The American

Drugless Practitioners (AADP). Her expertise of over 15 years in the wellness industry, includes identifying acid/alkaline balance in the blood through education and demonstration of the "New Biology ™".

She continued her wellness practice becoming certified in Light Therapy using The Chiren and enhancement with color light therapy. In her practice, she helps her clients understand the importance of food, air, water and sunshine and guides them to be proactive in their health concerns. She works through 3-6 month programs for both individuals and groups in addition to promoting wellness through a series of informative topics while guiding her clients to a healthier lifestyle with choices they learn to make.

Healing follows a natural approach, circulation, healthy blood, clean water and oxygen.

Helping People Achieve Optimal Health through education, knowledge, understanding and awareness.

Contact Information:

Email: Denise@findyourfountain.com

Website: www.findyourfountain.com

301 West Grove Street

Clarks Summit, PA 18411

570-561-5063

Luanne Pennesi, RN, MS

Individualized Consultations
Providing a Comprehensive Lifestyle Assessment

Luanne Pennesi, a registered nurse practicing for over 35 years in both conventional and integrative medicine, is the new rising star in the field of natural health, sharing information that motivates people to take back their personal power and lead happier more productive lives at ANY age.

Luanne's work has been called the missing link between gathering sometimes confusing, overwhelming and conflicting information about "new age" or "alternative" approaches to health and anti-aging and the practical application of real-time, commonsense, scientifically based information to help you take full control over your health and longevity and often save your own life naturally.

Having had an extensive clinical and administrative background in Adult medicine and Oncology (cancer) nursing, Luanne knows first hand the devastating effects of chronic stress, leading a toxic lifestyle, developing chronic illnesses and enduring the long term, debilitating side effects of many conventional medical therapies. She also has a solid background as a nursing leader, serving as a nurse administrator for 18 years at a major New York City Medical Center as well as the founder and executive director of one of the fastest growing wellness centers in the Tri-State area.

Luanne:"I believe that the technology and diagnostic wisdom of conventional medicine is essential to utilize, and I also believe that emergency medicine and reconstructive surgeries help people to live longer, more quality lives. What I object to is the arrogance of a system that does not honor time tested, scientifically documented therapies that do not originate from their sacred halls, those that they cannot assert political and fiscal control over. It is time we offered the public alternatives to many standard medical therapies that just plain don't help people to heal. I have witnessed people who have reversed dozens of conditions that conventional medicine has failed miserably at reversing in spite of the millions of dollars of research that go into studies controlled by the very pharmaceutical companies that are selling the drugs to suppress the symptoms that our bodies manifest in order to beg our attention."

Her extensive credentials and experience include:

- Masters of Science in Natural Health
- Nursing license in NY, NJ, Florida, California

- Certified Nurse AMMA therapist, which is a comprehensive and sophisticated Oriental diagnosis and massage therapy with acupressure point treatment
- Certified Neurolinguistic Healer
- Level IIB Healing Touch practitioner
- Founder of the Metropolitan Wellness Group, a NYC-based wholistic wellness center, which is now Metropolitan Medical HealthCare & Wellness. Luanne is now the Executive Director of the center as well as their premiere Lifestyle Counselor.
- She was the NYS coordinator for The American Holistic Nurses Association for 5 years.
- She was the Program Coordinator of Stress Management and Esteem Building for the Wholistic Nursing Programs at the New York College for Wholistic Health, Education and Research in Syosset, NY.
- She is trained in the use of high dose vitamin C and bio-oxidative therapies as well.
- She was recognized in "Who's Who Among Young American Professionals" in 1988 and "Who's Who in American Nursing" in 1994.

- A regular guest on local talk radio, Luanne co-hosted the radio program "The Tri-State Healing Hour" with Gary Null on WEVD in 1997 and "Creative Wellness" on WHPC from Nassau Community College in 1996 and 1997.
- In 2000, she hosted her own show, The Healing Hour, in Fort Lauderdale, Florida.
- She was a founding member and was a broadcast affiliate for The People's Network, a revolutionary television network devoted exclusively to providing motivational, instructional, inspiring and success-oriented programming.
- You can see her on Staten Island Cablevision's The Thinking Mind with George Stern and the Metro Channel's Health Styles with Mary Mucci.
- Luanne often shares the stage with health and nutrition expert Gary Null at his health support groups all around the country and assists him with updating his world famous, highly effective natural protocols for chronic illnesses.

Luanne is a dynamic, energizing individual who makes learning fun as she presents wholistic health concepts in a manner that is easy to understand and to integrate. To prove her authenticity, she personally lives the healthy, positive, adventurous life that she prescribes for others.

At Metropolitan Wellness my mission is to help others to create and maintain high levels of health, vitality and wealth which often includes the focused attention to one's current and past imbalances.

Areas of focus include:

- Physiology/physical body
- Mental/emotional body
- Physical environment/personal hygiene
- Spiritual self/bliss/peace of mind
- Spectrum of energy around the body, auras and chakras
- Constitution/genetic expressions

Programs by Luanne Pennesi

Getting Your Head on Straight: Understanding your mind and how to not lose it

Staying Healthy in an Ailing Economy

Living Authentically: How to be happy, healthy and financially free

Shift happens: How to create and manage change

Zen and the Art of Spring Cleaning

Andropause and Menopause- A natural approach

Mean, Lean vegetarian Cuisine ™

Dealing with Stress…and other stuff we can't control

SOULUTIONS™: How to relax and be inspired

Natural Approaches to Chronic Illness: Wholism and the use of Alternative therapies

NURSE POWER: How to start your own business, market yourself & earn extra money as an RN

Healthy, Functional Relationships start with YOU

Standing in Your Power- The fine Art of Mental Toughness, how to Communicate and how to Lead by example

Laugh your ass off: How to really have fun

Individual Consultations With Luanne Pennesi, RN, MS, Licensed in NY, CA, FL, NJ, PA

Why consult with Luanne? Because here is what you get:

Comprehensive Lifestyle Assessment

1. First we need to see what created your imbalances; ie, what are the risk factors that led to the diagnosis.
2. Next we need to ascertain the degree of toxicity you have accumulated in your body, your environment and your mind/thoughts/emotions and begin detoxifying on all levels.
3. Once that process has begun we integrate repairing/healing modalities on all 3 levels, and finally we rejuvenate and challenge the immune system.
4. Then you are placed on a maintenance protocol to keep the immune system strong

Individualized Healthy Lifestyle Protocol

- We start out with a 1 1/2 hour initial consultation either by phone or in person. I have offices in Coram, NY, Smithtown, NY, Glen Cove, NY, New York City, LA and Naples, Fla. The consultation includes a soon to be published workbook, over 100 pages long, individualized protocols, references, resources, referrals plus my comprehensive life/health assessment.

- Then I follow you once a week for 4 weeks then once a month for 5 months; you can contact me via phone or Internet with what you have accomplished what you are working on next, what changes you have experienced and any questions you have for me.
- I work as a part of your health team, which often includes your MD, both conventional and holistic, and any other practitioners such as chiropractors, colon hydrotherapists, acupuncturists, nutritionists, etc.

What you need to bring with you in writing, or e-mail to Luanne at <u>whnn@aol.com</u>**:**

1. What your diet is like
2. A list of medications and supplements you are taking
3. A brief medical history
4. A list of all the things you've always wanted to do in life but have not had the opportunity to do so far due to your life's circumstances
5. Name, address, phone number
6. E-mail address if you have one
7. Your age

Testimonials

May 2008

Hi Luanne,

Everything is good with me. I'm still juicing greens daily and it adds such a huge dimension to my wellbeing. I am for the most part completely medication free.

How many times can a person say THANKS? Your guidance has enabled me to regain a large part of myself.

Regards,
Marlene

April 2008

"I believe your life experiences, research, holistic studies and outlook on life has changed me and each and every person you encourage and touch with your work. I have learned so much from you."

Violeta Barias, lecture participant

"If you are ready to take control of your health and your life, you need sound advice, straight talk and an abundance of information from an authentic health and wellness professional, Luanne Pennesi will make you feel worthy of all that you will become on your journey toward ultimate health and happiness."

Deborah Fredericks, New Jersey

"Your workbook is probably the most information packed manual on lifestyle and health that I've ever seen. It is invaluable information and I know I will be using it for reference, inspiration, and for filling in gaps in my life and health. I am super happy that it has all of this combined: lifestyle, nutrition, inspiration, health, and so much more. It's like a manual for life. You have something here that is priceless."

Peter Alexander, Colorado Springs, CO

Contact Information:

Luanne Pennesi can be reached at her home office.

Phone: 631-504-6198

Email: whnn@aol.com

Website: www.metropolitanwellness.com

Chris Wark

An Inspirational Story

I was having some abdominal pain on and off for the better part of 2003, and being the typical male, I put it off. I thought it might be an ulcer and that it would eventually get better, but it didn't. It was kind of like the movie Groundhog Day. Every morning I would wake up feeling good, but several times a day I would get these brief flashes of pain in the afternoon and evening. Sometimes in the middle of the night. It wasn't a constant pain and didn't interfere with my life, but I was concerned. The next morning I would wake up feeling good again. Eventually the pain became so intense that I found myself balled up on the couch every night after dinner. Time to see a doctor.

After a series of inconclusive tests I was sent to a gastroenterologist for a colonoscopy. Turns out there was a golf ball sized tumor in my large intestine. Great. They did a biopsy and told me I had colon cancer. It was two weeks before Christmas 2003 and I was 26 years old. I was in shock. I couldn't believe this was my life. How did I end up with an old person's disease? I felt weak and pathetic. I was embarrassed and fearful, but I was reminded of these scriptures:

"And we know that God causes all things to work together for good to those who love God, to those who are called according to His purpose."
-Romans 8:28

"The righteous man may suffer many afflictions but the LORD delivers him from them all." -Psalm 34

"Trust in the LORD, and do not lean on your own understanding. In all your ways acknowledge HIm and He will make your paths straight."
-Proverbs 3:5

Even though I didn't understand why I was sick, I knew that God was in control.

Three weeks later I had surgery. They removed the tumor and a third of my colon. The cancer had spread to my lymph nodes. It was classified as Stage 3. They brought an oncologist into my room and he informed me that I would need 9-12 months of chemotherapy after I recovered from surgery.

The first meal they served me in the hospital after removing a third of my large intestine was a sloppy joe. I was starving. I hadn't eaten in three days, but I couldn't get down more than a few bites. I was relatively clueless about nutrition, but I instinctively knew that a sloppy joe was the last thing my body needed.

Before I checked out of the hospital I asked the surgeon, "Are there any foods I need to avoid?" He said, "Nah, just don't lift anything heavier than a beer." Not the advice I was expecting.

When we got home my wife and I prayed and asked God

that if there was another way besides chemotherapy that He would reveal it to us.

Two days later a book arrived on my doorstep, sent to me from a man in Alaska who I'd never met. He was a business acquaintance of my fathers.

That book was called "God's Way to Ultimate Health" by George Malkmus and it detailed how he beat colon cancer nearly 30 years earlier using natural methods including the raw vegan diet and juicing; without surgery or chemotherapy. I knew it was an answer to prayer. I realized that my nutrient deficient diet of artificial processed food, fast food, junk food, and factory farmed animal products was killing me. I started to do more research on the harmful nature of cancer therapies and discovered that chemotherapy destroys the immune system, makes cancer stem cells more aggressive, causes secondary cancers, and would likely make me infertile. That was when I decided against chemotherapy.

This decision was not well received by my wife and many family members. After intense family pressure I agreed to meet with an oncologist to hear what he had to say. He told me I had a 60% chance of living 5 years with conventional therapies. To me that wasn't much better than a coin toss. I asked him about alternative therapies. He looked me dead in the eye and said, "There are none. If you don't do chemo, you are insane... And I'm not saying this because I need your business". My wife and I left the clinic terrified. We sat in the car, held hands, cried and prayed.

The only people who supported me initially were my parents, even my wife wanted me to do chemotherapy. There was a tremendous amount of pressure to follow the doctor's orders and I was afraid of dying and looking like a fool for trying alternative therapies, but I knew God was leading me down a different path. He gave me courage and peace in the midst of all the uncertainty and opposition.

"For I know the plans I have for you," says the LORD, "plans to prosper you and not to harm you, plans to give you hope and a future."
-Jeremiah 29:11

I knew I wasn't taking care of myself and that there were massive radical changes I could make to my diet and lifestyle. So I decided to take responsibility for my health and recovery. And if that didn't work, chemo would be my last resort.

I radically changed my diet eating massive amounts of mostly raw fruits, vegetables, seeds and nuts with not animal products for 90 days. I drank 8 glasses of fresh vegetable juice every day for nearly two years. I did every alternative, holistic, non-toxic therapy I could find and afford including: Fasting, Vitamin C IVs, Rebounding, Immune boosting and detox supplements, Herbal Teas, Acupuncture, Structural Integration, Hydrotherapy, Saunas and more.

I found a local holistic nutritionist in Memphis who was a tremendous ally. He guided me along my health journey with nutritional recommendations additional supplements, therapies and diagnostic tests. After 90 days he added some clean organic meats and a more cooked food back into my diet. From there I maintained a 70-80% raw diet. And I continued to research on my own; reading all the information I could find about natural cancer therapies. I was determined to live. By taking control of my health and radically transforming my diet and lifestyle, I enabled my body to heal and become a place where cancer could not thrive.

December 2013 marked my 10-year "cancerversay" My wife and I have two beautiful daughters ages 5 and 9, I am still cancer-free and in the best shape of my life.
As I write this I am reminded of how good God is. How much he loves us and cares for us. I put my trust in Him, not in modern medicine. He led me in the path of healing and he will lead you too if you let Him.

"I sought the Lord and He answered me, and delivered me from all my fears."
-Psalm 34:4

Chris Wark
Memphis, TN

My mission is to share the information about nutrition and natural therapies that saved my life along with natural survivor stories like mine. **www.ChrisBeatCancer.com**

...don't get mad and don't cuss a body out mentally or in voice. This brings more poisons than may be rated by even taking foods that aren't good.

*~ **Edgar Cayce Reading 470-37***

Section III

Options addressing the Mind and Spirit

Why It Is Important to Address the Mind and Spirit

The body, mind and spirit go hand in hand. The research I found explains how you can have the perfect healthy diet yet still become ill. The body, mind and spirit must be addressed along with diet and lifestyle changes for true healing to be attained. Remember, emotions can change your body's chemistry. It is at this time you obviously need to address what is "bugging you" and imperative that you make necessary lifestyle adjustments to help counter act the chemistry changes made by your emotions.

Dad was on a morphine-like patch along with oral pain killers. The tumor grew into his small intestine creating a duodenal ulcer. Due to much pain the dosage of medication was increased. Dad was shriveling up like a raisin. The medication did not stop the pain. However, he was so "high" that he could not fight the pain anymore. Eventually the ulcer perforated the small intestine and he died within hours.

Although cancer can be painful there must be other ways to relieve pain without creating more dis-ease within the body.

We needed to help Dad relieve his pain. We performed

Hands on Healing and Reiki. This helped him tremendously. He looked forward to this on a daily basis.

As a spiritual family we realized, including Dad, himself, why his body took on this dis-ease. He was at a crossroad and pending retirement. He needed something to replace his family business that he spent almost 50 years of his life developing. With no resolution in site, his spirit was dimming.

Remember, THERE IS A PURPOSE FOR ALL! Find your passion in life. Listen to the inner voice whispering to you throughout your life that you have been ignoring. Take one step each day working toward your goal. DON'T GIVE UP!

Listed ahead are references providing spiritual support.

The Personal Transformation and Courage Institute

The Personal Transformation and Courage Institute is a non-profit educational organization founded to help people in life transitions to courageously fulfill their potentials. Since 2000, hundreds of people have found life-changing support through PTCI. The workshop courses from PTCI are designed to give participants a direct experience of their own courage to take the next step in personal transformation - physically, mentally, and spiritually.

The courses are not therapy but are instead a powerful set of exercises and experiences designed to awaken a new sense of oneself and one's place in life. The courses are focused on deeper self-awareness and ways of making a connection to courage, creativity, and vitality. Follow-up personal mentoring with the course leaders is also available. Most of the workshop courses are held in Fairfax and Virginia Beach, Virginia - but PTCI also offers courses in other locations. See the "Schedule" page on the web site for a list of course topics and venues. For more details about the variety of courses we offer at different levels of intensity, see the "Courses" page on the web site.

There is a wide variety of Basic Courses available from the Institute, each focused on some aspect of personal transformation. These Basic Courses are usually three-days (mornings and afternoons) with a group of 8 to 16 participants. Here are two example courses:

"Vision and Courage" Course

Walking the spiritual path requires that we see a vision for our lives and move toward that vision with purpose and courage. This course provides a conceptual framework from the readings of Edgar Cayce and the work of Rudolf Steiner for working with "visioning" in our lives. The course then draws upon non-intellectual experiential modalities including synchronicity exercises with the Zen tarot cards, energy constellations, active meditations, and mandala drawing to access insights, create the space in our daily lives, and open our hearts to the courage needed to live our Ideals. Participants experiment with learning how to say "no" to those energies that stand in the way of their Ideals, so they can say "yes" to their genuine soul yearnings and purpose.

"Awakening the Compassionate Heart" Course

No one can protect themselves or another from experiencing a broken or wounded heart. But we do have control over whether or not our hearts become bitter. This course assists the participants to gently and lovingly confront the vulnerability and woundedness of our hearts.

Through experiential exercises, students learn to be compassionate toward themselves so they can begin to heal those tender places in their hearts and find the gifts embedded in that woundedness.

Self-exploration through inquiry, synchronicity exercises with the Zen tarot cards, energy constellations, active meditations, and mandala drawing modalities are used to help students access the latent strength in the courageous and open heart.

Visit the PTCI web site for course dates and locations, or to contact the Institute about how you can enroll in a course. There is also an online video about the courses, plus a photo essay of what it's like to be at a course.

To see testimonials from PTCI students please go to the website.

Contact information:

The Personal Transformation and Courage Institute

Website: www.transformationANDcourage.org

Email: info@transformationANDcourage.org

Phone: 1-757-496-2961

Address: Mark Thurston, PO Box 914 Virginia Beach, VA 23451

The Art of Living Course

The Art of Living Course gives participants the practical knowledge and techniques to unlock their deepest potential and bring fullness to life. Whether happy and successful or feeling the stress of poor health, disappointments, or fear, every participant is cared for and comes away lighter, with effective techniques for releasing mental and physical stress and increasing his or her health, energy, peace, self-knowledge, awareness, and joy.

What you will learn

- **Practices** that heal and harmonize the body, mind, and spirit
- **Skills** for handling negative emotions and situations
- **Practical wisdom** for improving work and relationships
- **Insight** into the laws that govern the mind and emotions
- **Stretching** and **low-impact yoga** for health, circulation, and body stillness

Experience Peace of Mind

Much of the stress or limitations in life come from vacillating between regret about the past or worry about the future. And yet, the present is the only place that happiness can be experienced. A remarkable feature of the course is

131

that participants are able to re-discover the present moment — not as a concept but as a direct experience.

Simple Techniques for Daily Life

Participants leave with simple but powerful techniques they can practice every day, and an extraordinary weekly group practice is available in many areas. These practices are sacred treasures that grow in value over the years, helping the benefits continue to blossom in daily life.

Sudarshan Kriya: The masterpiece of the Art of Living Course is a powerful breathing-based technique called Sudarshan Kriya, or the healing breath. Sudarshan Kriya incorporates specific natural rhythms of breath to release stress and bring the mind to the present moment. The course also includes other breathing techniques, meditation, low-impact yoga, and skills for dealing effectively with challenging emotions and situations.

Several independent **studies** on the numerous mental and physical health benefits of the course have been published in international peer-reviewed journals and confirm what **participants commonly report.**

The Art of Living Course has been enjoyed by people of all traditions, religions, and walks of life, in universities, churches, governments, businesses, prisons, war zones, community rooms, and living rooms. The course is complete in itself and is also a foundation for other Art of Living programs.

Benefits of the Art of Living Course

The Art of Living Course teaches us how to have greater peace, energy and joy...for a lifetime. We have learned many skills at home and in school, but we have never been taught how to handle negative emotions like anger, sadness, fear etc. If we learn the skill to deal with our mind when these emotions arise, the quality of our lives can change significantly for the better. Through the power of the breath and ancient knowledge of the mind, the Art of Living course teaches us this skill.

Return to Joy

Our mind tends to vacillate between the past and the future. We are either regretting the past or anxious about the future. However as we all know living in the present moment is the route to joy. Our mind is such that we cannot control it in a direct manner. We cannot force it to be in the present moment. But we can influence our mind through the breath. "Take a deep breath" is an age-old recommendation for relaxation. The Art of Living course takes this effect of breath on our minds and applies it in a very precise and powerful manner through the Sudarshan Kriya technique. Practice of this technique can bring our mind effortlessly into the present moment. As this happens, we learn the ability to reduce the effects of negative emotions and return to our natural state of joy.

Restoring the Natural Rhythm

There is a rhythm in all parts of nature; the sun rises and sets with a particular rhythm, the tides rise and ebb with their own rhythm, our body wakes and sleeps with a certain rhythm. Similarly every emotion has a corresponding rhythm in the breath. In the Art of Living Course we use this link between our breath and our emotions to come closer to the rhythm of our natural Being.

There are five types of restlessness:

Sri Sri Ravi Shankar explains

1. The first type of restlessness is due to the Place you are in. When you move away from that place, the street or the house, you immediately feel better.
2. Chanting, singing, children playing and laughing can change this atmospheric restlessness. If you chant and sing, the vibration in the place changes.
3. The second type of restlessness is in the Body. Eating the wrong food or vata aggravating food, eating at odd times, not exercising, and overworking can all cause a **physical restlessness**. The remedy for this is exercise, moderation in work habits and going on a vegetable or juice diet for one or two days.

4. The third type of restlessness is **mental restlessness**. It is caused by ambition, strong thoughts, likes or dislikes. Knowledge alone can cure this restlessness. Seeing life from a broader perspective, knowledge about the Self and the impermanence of everything. If you achieve everything, so what?

5. After your achievement, you will die. Knowledge of your death or life, confidence in the Self, in the Divine, can all calm down the mental restlessness.

6. The fifth type of restlessness is rare. It is the **restlessness of the soul**. When everything feels empty and meaningless, know you are very fortunate. That longing and restlessness is the restlessness of the soul. Do not try to get rid of it.

Embrace it! Welcome it! Usually to get rid of it people do all sorts of things - they change places, jobs or partners, do this, do that. It seems to help for some time, but it does not last.

This restlessness of the soul alone can bring authentic prayer in you. It brings perfection, Siddhis and miracles in life. It is so precious to get that inner most longing for the Divine. Satsang, the presence of the enlightened one, soothes the restlessness of the soul.

The Power of Meditation

What is Meditation? Settling the surface mind is meditation. Living in the present is meditation. Relaxing deeply is meditation. When you are really happy, reposing in love, you are meditating. Meditation is that space when the thoughts have subsided, and the mind is in complete rest.

Why do we Meditate?

When we are tense, or when we cannot concentrate on the activity at hand, it is usually because too many thoughts are passing through our mind. When the mind settles down, it lets go of tension and stress and centers itself in the present moment. Daily practice of meditation enables you to gain an increased ability to focus and concentrate, as well as clarity of mind and expanded awareness. Meditation also removes past impressions, and provides relaxation and deep rest. The rest you gain in effortless meditation is deeper than the deepest sleep.

The Key to Meditating

Often meditation is associated with effort — an effort to not think. When a person sits to meditate, there may be so many thoughts to begin with. The key to reducing these thoughts and reaching the underlying meditative state is through the breath. Through specific, natural breathing techniques, it's possible to quiet the mind of thoughts, preparing it to slip easily into meditation.

Sudarshan Kriya Takes You to Meditation

The Sudarshan Kriya breathing technique, brought out by Art of Living Foundation Founder His Holiness Sri Sri Ravi Shankar, incorporates specific natural rhythms of breath that release stress, detoxify the body, and center the mind in the present moment, naturally bringing it to a meditative state. Quieting the mind and dissolving deep into meditation, this technique brings joy, peace, and a sense of belonging to oneself and others.

Sahaj Samadhi Meditation

Sudarshan Kriya leaves you in a state of meditation and helps you live it throughout the day. A specific technique called Sahaj Samadhi Meditation expands the conscious mind, and lets you dwell in that state, further culturing the nervous system to support that clarity, bliss, and awareness in daily activity. Sahaj Samadhi means "natural enlightenment," and is an effortless technique that expands the awareness and releases the stress that limits awareness and joy. While easy to learn and practice, it requires its own short course and individual instruction session to learn. It is the delicate art of not-doing. It brings a wholeness to life, and, together with Sudarshan Kriya, helps a person know who they really are, beyond their passing thoughts and feelings.

It is in every person's faculty to experience the benefits of a regular meditation practice and the Sudarshan Kriya breathing technique. Breath and meditation is the body's natural way to quiet the mind of thoughts, experience deep rest and energize and heal the entire system.

The Science of Breath

In a fast paced age where stress and depression are widespread, the toll of these on physical and mental health can be extremely high. Stress, anxiety and depression are known to be significant factors in the onset and progression of a wide spectrum of illnesses ranging from cancer and HIV-1 infection, to asthma and cardiovascular disease.

The goal of the International Art of Living Foundation is to provide people from all layers of society with practical and effective tools, derived from the ancient yogic science of breath, to alleviate stress, improve health and increase wellness. The Art of Living International Research and Health Promotion Center aims to promote timely and scholarly investigation on these practices as they relate to physical, social, and emotional wellbeing.

Sudarshan Kriya® and its accompanying practices (SK&P), taught by the Art of Living Foundation world-wide, are time-honored stress management/health promotion techniques whose health benefits are being validated by modern medical science.

Independent research has shown that SK&P significantly:

- Reduces levels of stress (reduce cortisol - the "stress" hormone)
- Supports the immune system
- Increases optimism
- Relieves anxiety and depression (mild, moderate and severe)
- Increases anti-oxidant protection
- Enhances brain function (increased mental focus, calmness and recovery from stressful stimuli)
- Enhances well-being and peace of mind

These simple, yet powerful breathing practices have a unique advantage: they are free from unwanted side-effects, can cut health care costs, and are easy to learn and practice in daily life.

We welcome research collaborations and suggestions from all interested parties.

Contact Information:

Art of Living Foundation

2401 15th Street NW
Washington DC 20009
Phone: 1-877-399-1008

Email: info@artofliving.org

Website: www.artoflivingnj.org

For your convenience there are centers located all over the world.

Dr. Gerald Epstein

Gerald N. Epstein, MD, is one of the foremost practitioners of integrative healthcare for healing and transformation. Trained as a Freudian analyst, he abandoned this direction in 1974 to study therapeutic uses of the imagination under the guidance of Madame Colette Aboulker–Muscat in Jerusalem. Since then, he has been a pioneer in the use of mental imagery for treating physical and emotional problems. As his work evolved over the years, he has become a leading exponent of the Western spiritual tradition and its application to healing and therapeutics.

Dr. Gerald Epstein - For the past 45 years, as a physician and teacher, I have taught thousands of people to transform their lives through the most powerful tool available – their minds. I share these methods with you so that you too can learn to:

- Heal yourself – physically, mentally and emotionally
- Become the master of yourself by reversing destructive habits
- Open yourself to Spirit

A cornerstone of my teaching is the use of <u>mental imagery</u> – sometimes called guided imagery or visualization. Imagery has been used for thousands of years by healers and wisdom keepers of many cultures to heal the sick, to benefit the community, and connect to the Divine. All my teachings aim to encourage and preserve your freedom.

I hope this will empower you to take charge of your life to create new realities and experiences for yourself.

Mental Imagery

What is mental or guided imagery?

Imagery is the mind thinking visually in pictures. There are many ways we can think. For example, we think logically with words and non–logically through image, intuition, etc. We think in images all the time, but may not be aware of it. For instance, when we choose a shirt we are already envisioning ourselves in it before we put it on. A basketball player envisions the shot before s/he shoots the ball. In fact, images form the structure of our inner life. For example, night dreams come in the form of images.

What types of situations can imagery be used for?

- Any physical, emotional, mental or social difficulty
- To manage the creative process
- To bring couples closer together
- To create harmony in the family

The only known area where it may not serve at first is in the case of schizophrenia. Otherwise, everything is possible.

What is the origin of "mental imagery?"

The use of mental imagery goes back to our most ancient sources. Thousands of years ago we find a clear depiction of this process in the experience of the prophet Ezekiel, who travels in an inward imaginal journey to the throne of God. In fact, in biblical times there were schools called

Sons of the Prophets in which these imaging techniques were taught. As time went on a tradition emerged called Chariot or Throne mysticism that became an important branch of western spiritual practice called Kabbalah, the word itself meaning "to receive." Eventually the Catholic Church took up these practices in the person of some well–known saints including: Hildegarde of Bingen, Ignatius of Loyola, Teresa of Avila, as main luminaries. At the time of the Renaissance, mental imagery was the major technique of medical practice for treating people with physical illness. The name of the technique associated with this direction was called "complexio."

In summary: mental imagery has a long, unabated, and distinguished history of which the above represents only a brief pinkie–nail sketch. In the twentieth century, mental imagery had begun to flourish more extensively in Europe and America, especially in the latter half. Such names as Robert Desoille (Directed Waking Dream), Hanscarl Leuner (Guided Affective Imagery), Carl Jung (Active Imagination), and most importantly, Mme. Colette Aboulker–Muscat (Waking Dream Therapy), stand out as seminal contributors. To this list I add my own as the American link of this great tradition.

Is there a difference between "mental imagery," "guided imagery," or "visualization"?

Although the terms are used interchangeably in common parlance, I prefer the name "mental imagery" to "guided imagery" because generally you do not need another human being to lead you through the process. While I initially provide imagery exercises, as you become proficient in this simple and powerful technique, spontaneous imagery will arise from within you. Likewise, "visualization" stresses the visual sense rather than the engagement of all your senses. It   usually bespeaks a conjuring up of something that you have experienced previously or know about in the world rather than a spontaneous discovery you make in the inner forum of consciousness.

Why do I only practice it for a minute or so each day?

Imagery is like a firework display. You need only a single match to ignite a cascade of fireworks: So for a micro input you get a macro response.

Like any medicine, you need to repeat it generally three times a day for 21 days. Twenty–one days is a natural cycle of the human body. Research has shown that it takes up to 21 days to break a habit.

How can imagery bring about change in our daily lives?

Our inner images reflect our beliefs about the world. These beliefs spark the birth of our outer reality. The images that we conceive and perceive internally manifest, or are birthed, externally in the world. As you practice imagery you can experiment and see if this is true for you.

How does imagery work in healing physical ailments?

As noted above imagery is the mind thinking in pictures. The mind and physical body are mirror images of each other; they are two sides of the same coin. What happens in one happens in the other. If you see yourself healing in your mind's eye, the healing takes place in your physical body as well.

Listed below are two exercises taken from my book, Healing Visualizations: Creating Health Through Imagery.

I call these exercises God's Hands and Lightning Hands.
Intention: To clean out cancer.
Frequency: Three times a day, up to 1 minute, for nine cycles of 21 days of use and 7 days off. (You can stop anytime during the imagery cycle if your condition has healed.)

Cancer is a disease fed by many sources: emotional (loss, grief depression); environmental (environmental contamination of water, air, food, and the effects of radiation exposure); social (breakdowns in our social familial, or business relationships); moral/ethical (errors in the integrity of our moral behavior). Becoming aware of these contributory elements is an extremely valuable step in promoting cancer healing. If you feel stymied in working these matters out for yourself, seek the help of a trained clinician who is accepting of these conditions as contributory factors in cancer. Don't feel any compunctions about seeking this help and, above all, do not feel guilty or intimidated if your physician does not agree with your decision to explore additional therapies. DO what you need to do. Your life comes first and foremost. Take authority for yourself.

Here are two general cancer-healing exercises that can be employed by anyone suffering from this disease. These exercises can be useful in ameliorating the overall condition. The first exercise is for those who have religious inclinations.

God's Hands

Close your eyes. Breathe out three times and see yourself
as being God's hands. Breathe out once. Seeing your hands
as the Almighty's, touch the place on and in the diseased
area, gently cleaning out all the dirt and contamination and
then putting in order what has been in disorder (for
example, weaving together the fibers of the wall of the
colon). Then, breathe out once and see your body in perfect
condition. Your face is happy and smiling and your brain is
working in the most adequate way. Like yourself, and see
yourself being washed by a light sunshower coming from
above. Be proud of the body you have constructed. Breath
out once, then open your eyes.

Lightning Hands

Close your eyes. Breathe out three times and see your
hands become lightning bolts. Enter your body with them
to the place of disease. Take out what is there as you inhale
quickly, then quickly remove the lightning hands, bringing
the diseased matter with them. Throw it all behind you.
Then see a small waterfall above you and bathe in it,
feeling thoroughly cleansed. Breath out once, then open
your eyes.

Choosing Life

Choosing life is what being alive is all about. When we
choose life via positive beliefs, we align ourselves with
rhythms, harmony, abundance, and grace of the universe.
Have absolutely no doubt about this. It is a promise that has
been made to us from the beginning.

Imagery is a positive belief system. It enables us to choose life. If such an opportunity for healing and salvation has been offered, why not take advantage of it?

A great sage, who was a dear close friend, gave me an incredible insight before her death. I had asked her to tell me the meaning of life. She said, "Become a law unto yourself". Because she had the gift for saying so much in so few words, I asked her if she could expand on that thought. She complied readily, and in her characteristically pithy manner she added: "Become your own authority." For me the statement was a revelation and was all that needed to be said. For you, I would add: Let your personal trouble be the starting point for taking charge of your life. Use imagery to help yourself become your own authority. Let your beliefs create your experience and say yes to life.

***

Dr. Epstein has published many books and audios including: Waking Dream Therapy, Healing Visualizations, Healing Into Immortality, Climbing Jacob's Ladder, The Natural Laws of Self Healing, and The Phoenix Process. His latest works are Kabbalah for Inner Peace and Emotional Mastery.

He maintains a private practice in NY and is an Assistant Clinical Professor of Psychiatry at Mount Sinai Medical Center in New York. Dr. Epstein founded and directs The American Institute for Mental Imagery (AIMI) where he trains clinicians and educates the public in imagery, dreams and the western spiritual tradition.

Contact Information:

Dr. Gerald Epstein, M.D.
351 East 84th St. Suite 10-D
New York, New York 10028, USA

Phone: 212-369-4080
Email: jerry@drjerryepstein.org
Website: www.drjerryepstein.org

__Innersource__

Eden Energy Medicine

Put Healing in Good Hands-- Your Own

Energy Medicine awakens energies that bring vitality, joy, and enthusiasm to your life – and greater health to your body, mind,and spirit! Balancing your energies balances your body's chemistry, regulates your hormones, helps you feel better, and helps you think better. It can be used to overcome illness, and it can be used to keep you strong and resilient. It is the medicine of the future, but it empowers you NOW to adapt and even flourish in the 21st century.

Top 4 Questions About Energy Medicine

1. How is Energy Medicine Practiced?

Energy Medicine heals the body by activating its natural healing energies; you also heal the body by restoring energies that have become weak, disturbed, or out of balance. It utilizes techniques from healing traditions such as acupuncture, yoga, kinesiology, and qi gong. Flow, balance, and harmony can be non-invasively restored and maintained within an energy system by tapping, massaging, pinching, twisting, or connecting specific energy points (acupoints) on the skin; by tracing or swirling the hand over the skin along specific energy pathways; through exercises or postures designed for specific energetic effects; by focused use of the mind to move specific energies; and/or by surrounding an area with healing energies.

2. How Does It Work?

Energy Medicine recognizes energy as a vital, living, moving force that determines much about health and happiness. In Energy Medicine, energy is the medicine, and energy is also the patient:

- You heal the body by activating its natural healing energies (energy as the medicine).
- You also heal the body by restoring energies that have become weak, disturbed, or out of balance (energy as the patient).

To overcome illness and maintain vibrant health, the body needs its energies to:

- Move and have space to continue to move— energies may become blocked due to toxins, muscular or other constriction, prolonged stress, or interference from other energies.
- Move in specific patterns—generally in harmony with the physical structures and functions that the energies animate and support. "Flow follows function."
- Cross over—at all levels, from the microlevel of the double helix of DNA, extending to the macrolevel where the left side of the brain controls the right side of the body and the right side controls the left.

- Maintain a balance with other energies—the energies may lose their natural balance due to prolonged stress or other conditions that keep specific energy systems in a survival mode.
- Conversely, when the body is not healthy, corresponding disturbances in its energies can be identified and treated.

3. Is Energy Medicine Spiritual?

Entering the world of your body's subtle energies is a bridge into the domain of your deepest spiritual callings and your eternal essence. While no particular belief system, allegiance, or religious affiliation is associated with Energy Medicine, many people find that energy work touches into the realms of soul and
spirit.

4. Can anyone do it?

Absolutely! Working with your energies is your birthright!

Donna Eden

For more than 35 years, Donna Eden has been teaching people how to work with the body's energy systems to reclaim their health and natural vitality. Her award-winning books are used as texts in hundreds of Energy Medicine classes worldwide.

Donna is among the world's most sought, most joyous, and most authoritative spokespersons for Energy Medicine. Her abilities as a healer are legendary. She has taught more than 80,000 people worldwide, both laypeople and professionals, how to understand the body as an energy system. Now you can study with her through her videos, DVDs, books, and other home study resources.

Able from childhood to clairvoyantly see the body's subtle energies, she not only works with those energies to further health, happiness, and vitality, she has made a career of teaching people who do not see energies how to work with them— joyfully and effectively.

Right Brain Definition of Energy Medicine: "Energy is your body's magic! It is your life force. You keep it healthy and it keeps you healthy. If you are sick or sad, shifting your energies feels good. When you care for these invisible energies, it makes your heart sing and your cells happy!"

- Donna Eden

David Feinstein

David Feinstein Ph.D., a clinical psychologist, has served on the faculties of The Johns Hopkins University School of Medicine, Antioch College, and the California School of Professional Psychology. He has contributed more than 80 articles to the professional literature and his eight books have won nine national awards, including the 2007 *USA Book News* Book of the Year in the Psychology/Mental Health Category (for *Personal Mythology*). He and his wife, Donna Eden, have built the world's largest and most vibrant organization teaching Energy Medicine. Their 900 certified practitioners are serving thousands of clients and teaching hundreds of classes in the U.S., Canada, Latin America, Europe, Asia, and Australia.

Left Brain Definition of Energy Medicine:
"Conventional medicine, at its foundation, focuses on the biochemistry of cells, tissue, and organs. Energy Medicine, at its foundation, focuses on the energy fields of the body that organize and control the growth and repair of cells, tissue, and organs. Changing impaired energy patterns may be the most efficient, least invasive way to improve the health of organs, cells, and psyche."

- David Feinstein, Ph. D

In summary, we named the organization "Innersource" in recognition that the *sources* for health and healing lie *within*. A universe of energies animates your body while deep inner wisdom can be called upon to navigate your way toward an increasingly meaningful and gratifying life.

To find a Eden Energy Medicine Certified Practitioner, please visit the directory on the website.

Contact Information:

Innersource
777 E Main St
Ashland, OR 97520
541-482-1800 x1
1-800-835-8332
Email: energy@innersource.net
Website: www.innersource.net

The ComedyCures Foundation

ABOUT SARANNE & THE COMEDYCURES FOUNDATION

The ComedyCures Foundation tickles funny bones! **We bring joy, laughter, and therapeutic humor programs to kids and grown-ups living with illness depression, trauma and disabilities**. Through large & small scale therapeutic comedy programs, we entertain and educate patients, families and caregivers about the power of a comic perspective and the benefits of laughter and positive emotions on the body, mind, and spirit. "Yes, laughter is great medicine!

The ComedyCures Foundation, a 501(c)3 human service organization, was launched from Saranne's chemo chair in 1999 as an outgrowth of her personal experience with the healing power of a comic perspective. Today, Saranne is cancer-free and has connected with more than 900,000 people at more than 975 **live events** rediscover their funny bones through her motivational, inspirational, laughter-rich performances and unique therapeutic productions.

Back in 1999, as a newly-diagnosed cancer patient, Saranne was greatly inspired by the writings of **Norman Cousins**, the pioneer of therapeutic humor. In 2007, Saranne had the honor of meeting three generations of the Cousins' family and sharing the therapeutic legacy of The ComedyCures Foundation.

Some other highlights of her incredible journey with ComedyCures include: The award-winning LaughingLunch events in New York City plus other programs in hospitals, orphanages, shelters, camps for ill kids, senior homes, and military bases around the world. **Saranne gave the first closing TEDx talk at The United Nations. In addition to also producing the first comedy event at The United Nations, she taught the first therapeutic humor workshop at The World Health Organization in Geneva. Saranne also hosted the first Mobile Health Conference for The First Ladies from around the world with The UN and WHO.** Saranne has collaborated with The US Marines and and other military. She also produced and hosted the first therapeutic entertainment reunion on Broadway for the families impacted by September 11th with Rotary International.

Saranne created "ComedyCures' LaughingLunch Break" which was featured daily on 1010 Wins Radio, bringing family-friendly humor to millions each week with the talent of over 100 ComedyCures' comedians. She then went on to launch and host "ComedyCures' LaughTalk Radio" live each week on AM970 The Apple in NYC.

Saranne and her work at ComedyCures.org have been featured in many books including Oprah's "Live Your Best Life". Saranne is featured as Oprah's first "Hero". Most recently, Saranne (and Dr. Kelly Turner) **launched the book "Radical Remission" on the Dr. Oz Show. "Radical Remission" features Saranne's miracle story and strategies for beating stage IV cancer, including utilizing the power of humor, laughter and positive emotions.**

Saranne is a stage IV cancer survivor, with no visible disease, and a world-renowned mind/body and therapeutic humor/laughter expert. Saranne resides in Bergen County, New Jersey but travels worldwide for ComedyCures' programs. **These award-winning**

programs are made possible by the hundreds of talented comedians and performers who collaborate with Saranne and our dedicated ComedyCures' staff.

Our Mission

Through private and corporate donations, and the goodwill and humor of the comedy industry, it is our mission to entertain and educate kids and grown-ups living with illness, their families, and medical caregivers about the benefits of laughter and a comic perspective on the mind, body, and spirit.

The ComedyCures Vision

Through our innovative, joy-filled programs and live-events, ComedyCures provides people living with illness the opportunity to integrate joy, laughter and comedy into each day.

Contact Information:

The ComedyCures Foundation

Website: www.ComedyCures.org

Email: info@ComedyCures.com

201-227-8410 & 888-300-3990

122 E Clinton Ave

Tenafly , NJ 07670

http://www.facebook.com/comedycures

Toni Kimble

http://www.twitter.com/comedycures

http://www.youtube.com/comedycures

LifeParticle Collaborative Healing

All of us and everything around us are made of elementary particles of energy. Not only is your body made of these particles, which author Ilchi Lee has dubbed LifeParticles, but so is your consciousness. When you view the world as LifeParticles through meditation, you take on the consciousness of that fundamental level. It's one of oneness, vastness, and limitless creative potential—the consciousness that has been achieved by meditation masters for centuries. With that consciousness, you can use LifeParticles, and what you picture becomes reality with the added power of your focused action. You are naturally a creator, says author Ilchi Lee. It's who you are. Lee brings the ultimate meditation state of the masters to you in a simple and accessible way. LifeParticle Meditation provides targeted visualization techniques for waking up your mind's abilities and making the changes you want in your life. Rather than being dragged by life's inevitable flow of change, the meditation allows you to understand, manage, and direct that flow. Join Ilchi Lee and thousands of other LifeParticle Meditation practitioners in using LifeParticles to: * improve your health * strengthen your relationships * make better choices * give and receive more love * experience profound self-transformation * manifest your dreams and desires * help society and the planet based on a lifetime of meditation experience. With examples from the realms of science and spirituality and stories from practitioners of LifeParticle Meditation around the world, Ilchi Lee opens up for you a new world of LifeParticles—a world of wonder, creativity, love, and peace.

159

There is also LifeParticle Collaborative Healing Circles. This life energy can be sent and received between others to impart healing.

If you have access to YouTube, you will find an amazing story of a woman who had a brain tumor. Her father was very instrumental incorporating LifeParticle Collaborative Healing which has been very beneficial. The video can be viewed on the LifeParticle Show at *www.youtube.com/watch?v=uUGmcMxR_0Q*.

Creator of LifeParticle Meditation, Ilchi Lee is a respected educator, mentor, author and innovator who has devoted himself to developing the awakened brain and teaching energy principles through numerous mind-body-spirit practices. He has penned thirty-four books, including the *New York Times* bestseller, *The Call of Sedona: Journey of the Heart*.

To learn more about LifeParticle Meditation from an experienced instructor, please find a nearby Dahn Yoga or Body + Brain Holistic Yoga Center. LifeParticle principles and meditation are taught at over 1,000 locations worldwide, including 120 centers in the United States. In addition to LifeParticle Meditation, they offer group classes and individual sessions in meditative movement and breathing, as well as personal growth workshops.

Contact information:

Dahn Yoga
Website: www.dahnyoga.com
877-477-YOGA

Body + Brain Holistic Yoga Centers
Website: www.bodybrain.com
480-664-2194

For online videos and articles:
Website: www.changeyourenergy.com

Section IV

Your Teeth!

<u>Your Teeth!</u>

I came across some research that peaked my curiosity. Our mouth and teeth play such an important role to our health and wellbeing.

In this chapter you will find informative companies addressing Root Canals, Amalgam (Mercury) fillings, getting tested for chemical sensitivity materials that would be used in your mouth and Holistic Dentistry.

Price-Pottenger Nutrition Foundation

Dr. Weston A. Price (1870-1948), a Cleveland dentist, has been called the "Isaac Newton of Nutrition." In his search for the causes of dental decay and physical degeneration that he observed in his dental practice, he turned from test tubes and microscopes to unstudied evidence among human beings. Dr. Price sought the factors responsible for fine teeth among the people who had them–isolated nonindustrialized people.

The world became his laboratory. As he traveled, his findings led him to the belief that dental caries and deformed dental arches resulting in crowded, crooked teeth and unattractive appearance were merely a sign of physical degeneration, resulting from what he had suspected– nutritional deficiencies.

Price traveled the world over in order to study isolated human groups, including sequestered villages in Switzerland, Gaelic communities in the Outer Hebrides, Eskimos and Indians of North America, Melanesian and Polynesian South Sea Islanders, African tribes, Australian Aborigines, New Zealand Maori and the Indians of South America. Wherever he went, Dr. Price found that beautiful straight teeth, freedom from decay, stalwart bodies, resistance to disease and fine characters were typical of primitives on their traditional diets, rich in essential food factors.

Dr. Price conducted extensive research into the destructive effects of root canals, detailed in his two-volume work

Dental Infections *Oral & Systemic* and *Dental Infections & the Degenerative Diseases.* His conclusions, ignored by the orthodox dental establishment for over 50 years, are gaining renewed acceptance as holistic practitioners are discovering that the first step to recovery from degenerative disease often involves removal of all root canals in the patient's mouth.

The principles of holistic dentistry, based on the research of Weston Price and Francis Pottenger, are as follows:

- Eat nutrient-dense whole foods, properly grown and prepared.
- Avoid root canals. If you have root canals that you suspect are causing disease, have them removed by a knowledgeable dentist.
- Avoid mercury (amalgam) fillings. If you have amalgam fillings, have them removed by a holistic dentist who specializes in mercury filling replacement.
- Orthodontics should include measures to widen the palate.

Extract teeth only when necessary, and then in such a way as to avoid leaving the jaw bone with cavitations, which can be focal points of infection.

Root Canal Dangers

DNA Studies Confirm Dr. Weston Price's Century-Old Findings

Toxic dental materials have created much havoc in the dental profession, as well as in patient health, for nearly two centuries. Dental mercury fillings, nickel crowns (especially in children, called "chrome crowns"), root canals and cavitations have been the target of concern for a long time.

Dental mercury was first exposed as a health-compromising product in 1840. The dental profession finally overcame the perception that putting toxic mercury in the mouth might be detrimental to human health; organized dentistry still considers the current fillings containing 50 percent mercury as "state of the art."

The toxicity of root canals was disclosed by Mayo's Clinic and Dr. Weston Price jointly back in about 1910. Close to a century ago. Price's textbook on root canals, published in 1922, upset the dental associations at that time, and still does today. The American Dental Association (ADA), denies his findings and claims that they have proven root canals to be safe; however, no published data from the ADA is available to confirm this statement- statements, but no actual research.

My attention was drawn to the increase in autoimmune disease after the high-copper amalgams of 1975 were initiated as "state of the art" fillings, which ADA claimed released no mercury. On the contrary, studies from Europe[1] found that the high-copper amalgams released fifty times more mercury than previous amalgam!

In watching these changes regarding the onset of autoimmune disease, I noticed a blip in the statistics—an increase in amyotrophic lateral sclerosis (ALS or Lou Gehrig's disease) in 1976.

The actual number of cases of multiple sclerosis increased tremendously, from an average of 8800 per year during the period 1970 to 1975, to an increase of up to 123,000 in one year. That year being 1976, the birth date of high-copper amalgams.

ROOT CANAL HAZARD

Is mercury the only dental hazard that can create conditions favorable to autoimmune diseases? No. There are bacteria in root canals that favor destruction of the nervous system and many other systems, resulting in the creation of autoimmune reactions.

What is the common denominator? The formation of a hapten. A hapten is a small molecule that can elicit an immune response only when attached to a large carrier such as a protein; the carrier may be one that also does not elicit an immune response by itself. In general, only large molecules, infectious agents, or insoluble foreign matter can elicit an immune response in the body.

Healthy cells have a code imprinted on them. It is called the Major Histo-compatibility Complex (MHC). This is your personal code called "self." Your body considers other code or alteration of this code to be "non-self." The immune system is trained to kill and eliminate any "non-self" invaders.

If an atom of mercury attaches to a normal healthy cell, a hapten is formed and the immune system immediately identifies that cell as "nonself." The immune system then proceeds to kill the contaminated cell. If mercury attaches to a nerve cell, the result is a neurological disease, such as multiple sclerosis, Lou Gehrig's disease, seizures or lupus. If mercury attaches to a binding site on a hormone, that endocrine function is altered. Mercury can attach to almost any cell in the body and create autoimmune diseases in those tissues.

Lately, it has become evident that toxins from anaerobic bacteria have the same ability to create non-self autoimmune diseases by interfering with the MHC. This is the project that Dr. Price began to study a century ago. Resistance from organized dentistry was the same then as it is today. Price wondered why dentistry was considered a "health" profession.

Price was concerned about the pathological bacteria found in nearly all root canal teeth of that time. He was able to transfer diseases harbored by humans from their extracted root canal teeth into rabbits by inserting a fragment of a root canal root under the skin in the belly area of a test rabbit. He found that root canal fragments from a person who had suffered a heart attack, when implanted into a rabbit, would cause a heart attack in the rabbit within a few weeks. Transference of heart disease could be accomplished 100 percent of the time. Some diseases transferred only 88 percent of the time, but the handwriting was on the wall.

Dr. Price discovered that root canals had within them bacteria capable of producing many diseases. They had no place in the body. Which is more important? The life of the tooth or the life of the patient? This is still the primary argument facing us today.

ROOT CANALS AND NEUROLOGICAL DISEASE

Considering the difficulty of culturing anaerobic bacteria, it was hard to identify them with 1920s technology. Most of the bacteria reported by organized dentistry at that time were aerobes of unknown significance. Today, with DNA analysis available, anaerobic bacteria (the dangerous kind) can be identified whether dead or alive by the presence of their tell tale DNA signatures.

Let's go back to the graphs of ALS up through the year 2000. Note an increase in 1976 and another increase in slope in 1991. In 1990, the dental association "suggested" that dentists perform thirty million root canals per year by the year 2000. Dentists accomplished that goal by 1999. As

I understand it, the bar has now been raised to sixty million per year.

The unexplained increase in MS (8800 to 123,000) coincided with the advent of high copper amalgams. The increase in ALS in the same year is suggestive of the same cause. ALS also increased in 1991 as more root canals were performed. Statistical coincidence?

The goal of dentistry is to save teeth. Root canals allow dentists to maintain many teeth for years instead of extracting them. But is this goal appropriate considering the biological expense exposed with DNA research? What is more important? To save the life of the tooth or that of the patient?

HAVENS FOR BACTERIA

Dr. Price, while head of research for the now-defunct National Dental Association, took one thousand extracted teeth and reamed them out as dentists normally do, prior to filling the canals with wax. Price sterilized the canals with forty different chemicals far too toxic to be used in a live human situation; he wanted to see whether the canals could be permanently sterilized. After forty-eight hours, each tooth was broken apart, and cultured for the presence of bacteria. Nine hundred ninety out of one thousand cultured toxic bacteria just two days after treatment with chemicals designed to make the tooth sterile. Where did these bacteria come from?

An overview of the structure of a tooth shows the outer layer, known as enamel, the second layer, known as dentin, and the inner portion, known as the pulp chamber, where the nerve lives. On the outside of the tooth is what is called the periodontal ligament. Teeth are not attached directly to bone. Fibers come out of the tooth and intertwine with fibers coming out of the bone, and they unite to form what is called the periodontal ligament.

The second layer of the tooth, the dentin, is not really solid but composed of tiny dentinal tubules. In a front tooth, if all these tubules were attached end to end, they would reach over three miles. Note that the tubules have adequate space to house many thousands of bacteria. This is where the bacteria were hiding in the thousand teeth Price tested. From the dentin tubules, bacteria can migrate either into the pulp chamber, where space is left as the gutta percha—a natural form of rubber used to fill the space inside the cleaned-out root—shrinks upon cooling, rebounding from the force applied to push the wax down the canal, and losing the liquid portion or into the periodontal ligament where a plentiful supply of food awaits them.

A tooth has one to four major canals. This fact is taught in dental school, but never mentioned are the additional "accessory canals." Price identified as many as seventy-five separate accessory canals in a single central incisor (the front tooth).

There is no way that any dental procedure can reach into these accessory canals and clean out the dead tissue. This necrotic tissue creates a home for multiple bacterial infections outside the tooth in the periodontal ligament. With added food supply from this area, the anaerobic bacteria can multiply and their toxins can contribute to the onset of disease.

Of course, the root apex (terminal end) is the primary area of concentration of infection. Even though this may be the last area to show infection, dentistry generally considers a tooth sterile unless areas of bone resorption show up on X-ray. Upon cooling and shrinking of the gutta percha, space is left at the apex in which bacteria can thrive, where neither white blood cells of the immune system, nor antibiotics can reach them.

TOXIC MICROORGANISMS

Our first DNA studies examined bacteria retrieved from crushed root tips. We can identify eighty-three different anaerobic bacterial species with DNA testing. Root canals contain fifty-three different species out of these eighty-three samples. Some are more dangerous than others, and some occur frequently, some occasionally. Selecting those that occur more than 5 percent of the time, we found:

Capnocytophaga ochracea
Fusobacterium nucleatum
Gemella morbillorum
Leptotrichia buccalis
Porphyromonas gingivalis

Of what significance are these? Four affect the heart, three the nerves, two the kidneys, two the brain and one the sinus cavities. Shouldn't we question the wisdom of supplying a haven for these microbes so close to our brain and circulatory system? Does this information validate the claims of "sterile" root canals?

Dentists claim they can "sterilize" the tooth before forcing the gutta percha wax down into the canal. Perhaps they can sterilize a column of air in the center of the tooth, but is that really where the problem is? Bacteria wandering out of the dentinal tubules is what Price was finding, and what we were finding in the crushed tooth samples. But does the problem end there? Hardly.

Just out of curiosity, we tested blood samples adjacent to the removed teeth and analyzed them for the presence of anaerobic bacteria. Approximately 400 percent more bacteria were found in the blood surrounding the root canal tooth than were in the tooth itself. It seems that the tooth is the incubator. The periodontal ligament supplies more food, therefore higher concentration of bacteria.

But the winner in pathological growth was in the bone surrounding the dead tooth. Looking at bacterial needs, there is a smorgasbord of bacterial nutrients present in the bone. This explains the tremendous increase in bacterial concentration in the blood surrounding the root canal tooth. Try sterilizing that volume of bone.

Apparently, the immune system doesn't care for dead

substances, and just the presence of dead tissue will cause the system to launch an attack. Infection, plus the autoimmune rejection reaction, causes more bacteria to collect around the dead tissue. Every time a person with a root canal bites down, these bacteria are flushed into the blood stream, and they start looking for a new home. Chemotaxis, or the chemical attraction of a specific bacteria for a specific tissue, assists the anaerobes in finding new quarters in the heart, nervous system, kidney, brain, etc., where they will perform their primary damage.

Many of the bacteria in the surrounding bone are present in far more than 50 percent of the samples tested. Streptococcus mutans was found in 92 percent of the blood samples. It can cause pneumonia, sinusitis, otitis media, meningitis and tooth decay.

Streptococcus mitis was found 92 percent of the time. This microbe attacks the heart and red blood cells. It is a rather hearty bug, for it went to the moon (hiding in a camera) on an unmanned expedition, stayed there over two years in an environment without atmosphere, exposed to temperatures of 250 degrees Fahrenheit during the day, minus 250 in the shadow. Upon returning to Earth with the astronauts of Apollo 12, over two years later, this microbe was still alive.[10] In humans, S. mitis binds to platelets and is involved in the pathogenesis of infective endocarditis. Want this guy living in your dead root canal tooth?

Of the top eight bacteria in the blood adjacent to root canal teeth, five affect the heart, five the nervous system, two the kidney, two the liver, and one attacks the brain sinus, where they kill red blood cells Of these, *Prevotella intermedia* (present in 76 percent of the samples) attacks heart, kidney and sinus; *Strep intermedius* (present in 69 percent of the samples) attacks heart, nerves, lungs, liver and brain.

DNA examination of extracted root canals has shown bacterial contamination in 100 percent of the samples tested. This is quite the opposite of official claims that root canals are 97 percent successful. Do they need a new definition of success?

CAVITATIONS

Cavitations are the next big problem that result from dental procedures. Cavitations are areas of unhealed bone left over after a tooth extraction.

Dentists are generally taught to remove a tooth and leave the periodontal ligament in the socket, a procedure which would be like delivering a baby and leaving the placenta in the uterus.

These socket areas with the ligament left in place rarely heal. After tooth removal, a cap of about 2 millimeters (one sixteenth of an inch) covers the extraction site, leaving a hole the size of the root of the tooth behind. In records of five thousand surgical debridements (cleaning) of cavitations, only two were found to be healed.[14] When the periodontal ligament is left in the bone, the body senses that the tooth is still there, and the order for healing is canceled. These holes are lined with many of the same bacteria found in root canal sockets, but actually more different species. Whereas root canal teeth contain up to fifty-three different species of bacteria, cavitations yield up to eighty-two of the eighty-three we test for.

Of the five most frequently present bacteria found in cavitations, three affect the heart, two the nervous system and one the kidneys and lungs. They are as follows:

Streptococcus mutans (occurrence 63 percent of the samples), affects the nervous system, can cause pneumonia, sinusitis, otitis media and meningitis. It has also been blamed for causing dental decay in teeth, but this may be more the result of the fluid flow pulling bacteria into the tooth than actual active invasion by the bacteria.

Porphyromonas gingivalis (occurring in 51 percent of the samples), damages the kidney, alters integrity of endothelial lining of blood vessels, and induces foam cells from macrophages, contributing to atherogenesis. It contains proteases that lyse red blood cells and extract nutrients (primarily iron) from the red blood cells. This action is called porin forming, which can destroy red blood cells rapidly. (By the way, *P. gingivalis* can both up and down regulate about five hundred different proteins critical to maintaining our normal biochemical actions.)

Candida albicans (present in 44 percent of the samples), in its yeast form is beneficial in the process of demethylation of methyl-mercury as well as its ability to destroy pathogenic bacteria in the intestinal tract. When converted into the fungal form by a shift in pH in the digestive system, candida can penetrate the intestinal wall, leaving microscopic holes that allow toxins, undigested food particles, bacteria and other yeasts to enter the blood stream. This condition is sometimes referred to as Leaky Gut Syndrome, which can lead to environmental intolerances.

Prevotella intermedia (occurrence rate of 44 percent) has as its primary concern coronary heart disease (CHD). *P. intermedia* invades human coronary artery endothelial cells and smooth muscle cells. It is generally located in atheromatous plaques. Cellular invasion of cardiac muscle is central to the infective process.[11]

ANTIBIOTICS

So, if all these diseases of "unknown etiology," that is, of unknown origin, are the result of bacterial invasion, why not just flood the body with antibiotics? They kill bacteria, don't they? Ever hear of someone who was sick, was given antibiotics, and then got even worse? Most of us have heard the story. Perhaps the following information explains what happens in these cases, and why antibiotics cannot be used in infections of this nature.

Most antibiotics are "bactericidal"—think suicidal, or homicidal. Antibiotics kill. But this is not the same type of killing that John Wayne was noted for. When he fired at the bad guy, the bad guy fell over dead. Was then presumed to be buried. But when bactericidal antibiotics kill a bacterium, the bacterium explodes.

The fragments are not eliminated immediately, for each piece is a lipopolysaccharide called endotoxin.[12] By way of contrast, exotoxins are the toxic chemicals that are released by pathogenic bacteria, and endotoxins are toxic entities (fragments of the original bacteria) that are the result of the bacterial explosion caused by the antibiotic. Endotoxins present a huge challenge to the immune system, for now, instead of facing one bacterium, it has to process and eliminate perhaps one hundred endotoxins. With dozens of bacteria to confront from each single root canal or cavitation, no one antibiotic can kill all of them, and if there were one, the resulting dead bacterial corpses would overwhelm the body and produce either greater disease or death.

Broad spectrum antibiotics cannot be used for this reason. Sometimes even one capsule of antibiotic produces more problems than the immune system can tolerate. Plus, of course, it takes only two or three capsules to completely sterilize the gut of its four or more pounds of friendly bacteria.[13] Antibiotics are far more powerful and potentially devastating than I ever thought they were. Antibiotics should be used with ultra caution, not routinely given for ten days or so after oral surgery, "just in case."

There are other ways to get these microbes under control, and several are being tested at this time. It is advantageous to have intravenous vitamin C and occasionally a non-killing antibiotic is added to this solution. This combination does reduce the challenge to the immune system, but, overall, root canals represent the rock-and-hard-place situation.

Leave the root canal or cavitation in the body, and there is the potential of creating an unwanted autoimmune or degenerative disease that could be life threatening. Toxins and bacteria can both leak from these contamination sites wreaking havoc with a person's cardiovascular, endocrine, nervous and immune systems. The public needs to be informed, so they can make educated choices in the trade-off between toxic convenience and health.

Removing the offending tooth presents problems that must be confronted, or other problems can be induced—problems not as dangerous as the continuous bacterial spill, but ones that need to be avoided if possible. In order to allow the immune system to focus on healing, all other offending dental materials should be removed (mercury, copper, implants, tattoos and nickel crowns) so that the immune system can deal with the bacterial challenge instead of the bacteria plus toxic metals. Nutrition should be calculated from the aspect of the blood chemistries commensurate with one's ancestral diet and in line with the dietary principles formulated by Dr. Price. Recovery from a root canal is complicated, but your patient's life is worth salvaging.

These studies in DNA analysis of bacteria in root canals and cavitations confirm the fact that Dr. Weston Price, despite being one century ahead of his colleagues, was absolutely correct in determining that bacteria-laden root canals have no place in the body of people interested in their health. This toxic waste spill can be stopped, but not with the assistance of dental associations, which continue to insist that the procedure of root canals is perfectly safe. The recent increase in suggested quota up to sixty million root canals per year is not in the best interest of their patients, nor can that action do anything but increase health costs for the innocent patient.

Price was right. Root canals are not worth the price.

BACTERIA LURKING IN ROOT CANALS

Let's look at five major bacterial species lurking in root canals more closely, keeping in mind that these are only five of the fifty-three that are routinely found in root canal teeth.

Capnocytophaga ochracea: Found in brain abscesses associated with dental source of infection. Causes human disease in the central nervous system. Also related to septicemia and meningitis.

Fusobacterium nucleatum: Produces toxins that inhibit fibroblast cell division and wound healing processes. Causes infection in the heart, joints, liver and spleen.

Gemella morbillorum: Linked to acute invasive endocarditis, septic arthritis and meningitis.

Leptotrichia buccalis: Reduces the number of neutrophils (a critically important white blood cell), thus lowering immune competence.

Porphyromonas gingivalis: Destroys red blood cells by drilling holes (porins) in them, causing the cell to "bleed to death." Low red cell counts that do not recover after dental revision are frequently responding to the porin activity of this microbe. *P. gingivalis* also alters the integrity of the endothelial lining of blood vessels, which leads to inflammation and bleeding in the inner lining of blood vessels. This is the key step in formation of atherogenesis that leads to heart attacks. *P. gingivalis* can change friendly bacteria into pathogens.

Please visit these informative sites:

Nutrition and Physical Degeneration:
http://ppnf.org/product/books-1/nutrition-and-physical-degeneration/ and *Root Canal Cover-Up:*
http://ppnf..org/product/books-1/root-canal-cover-up/

Contact information:

Price-Pottenger Nutrition Foundation

Website: www.ppnf.org

1-800-366-3748
619-462-7600

Holistic Dental Association

History

In 1978, concerned and dedicated dentists came together to share their common interest in treatment modalities that were not included in dental school curriculum. Some of these modalities were very new and others were very old; the one thing that they shared in common was they offered additional options for treatment. These dentists wished to establish an organization that would provide a forum for the development and sharing of health promoting therapies. The shift from the dentist's emphasis solely on dental procedures to a consideration of the attitudes and feelings of the patient and the dentist has occurred. The primary goal of the Holistic Dental Association, to teach and to learn, has not changed since the founding members first met.

In recent years, more and more individuals are assuming greater responsibility for their own health. There is a dawning awareness that good health is more than the absence of disease. In this regard, the Holistic Dental Association has assumed a primary obligation to provide information and guidance to those persons seeking to participate in their own health care and to help in the continuing education of practitioners who have a desire to expand their knowledge and awareness.

Contact information:

Holistic Dental Association

305-356-7338

Website: www.holisticdental.org

1825 Ponce de Leon Blvd. #148

Coral Gables, FL 33134

International Academy of Biological Dentistry and Medicine

The IABDM is a network of dentists, physicians and allied health professionals committed to caring for the whole person – body, mind, spirit and mouth.

We are dedicated to advancing excellence in the art and science of biological dentistry. We encourage the highest standards of ethical conduct and responsible patient care.

What Is Biological Dentistry?

Biological dentistry is concerned with the whole body effects of all dental materials, techniques and procedures.

It is fluoride-free, mercury-free and mercury-safe. Individualized testing for biocompatibility of dental materials is a must.

It insists that all clinical practice be designed of components that sustain life or improve the patient's quality of life.

For the word "biological" refers to life.

Clinical awareness and science show us that what happens in the mouth is reflected in the body, and what happens in the body is reflected in the mouth. The complex, dynamic relationships of oral and systemic health within the context of the whole person are inseparable.

Biological dentistry unites the best clinical practices and technologies of Western dental medicine with a wide array of practices beyond its horizon.

Biological dentists may be general dentists, periodontists, orthodontists, oral surgeons or pedodontists. They also have extensive training in dental toxicology and specific modes of healing, including Traditional Chinese Medicine (TCM), Ayurveda, herbology, homeopathy, iridology and energy medicine.

While it may be impossible to construct an authoritative list of protocols followed by the "typical" biological office, all share a common paradigm: treating causes of symptoms rather than symptoms toward the goal of restoring and sustaining health.

We also share a deep and constant belief in the Hippocratic dictate First, do no harm.

Biological dentistry is conservative dentistry. The aim is to be minimally invasive yet appropriately active.

Please view this informative video that explains how dentistry can impact the immune system-http://drdawn.net/learning-center/video/.

To find a practitioner please visit the website.

Contact Information:

281-651-1745

Email: drdawn@drdawn.net

Website: www.IABDM.org

19122 Camellia Bend Circle
Spring, Texas 77379

Clifford Materials Reactivity Testing

Clifford Materials Reactivity Testing (CMRT) is a laboratory screening process used to help identify existing sensitivity problems to various chemical groups and families of compounds in an individual patient. This process is currently being implemented in the CMRT Dental and Orthopedic panels. After a patient's test panel has been completed, the patient's reactivity test results are compiled in a report.

Dental Materials Screening Panel

Screening for systemic sensitivities to more than 15600 trade-named products and 94 chemical groups and families of dental products.

Contact Information:
Office: (719)550-0008
Fax: (719) 550-0009

Email: wjclifford@ccrlab.com

Mailing Address:
Clifford Consulting & Research Inc.
P.O. Box 50318
Colorado Springs CO. 80949

Street Address
Clifford Consulting & Research Inc.
4775 Centennial Blvd.
Suite 112
Colorado Springs CO.
USA

<u>Amalgam (Mercury) Fillings</u>

<u>Quicksilver Scientific</u>

Quicksilver Scientific is an analytical laboratory that specializes in mercury speciation analysis. The company is founded on advanced, patented technology that is completely scaleable and automated. This means Quicksilver's methods can easily handle various sample quantities. This also means that the Quicksilver method requires less labor, which in turn lowers the cost of analysis. Previously, this type of analysis was unaffordable (their panel would cost over $600).

The Product

Mercury speciation analysis is a process that separates and measures different forms of mercury. The Quicksilver method utilizes superior chemistries to provide the best accuracy and precision in the industry.

THE QS MERCURY TRI-TEST: A COMPLETE ANALYTICAL SOLUTION

Quicksilver Scientific's Tri-Test is the only clinical testing suite that measures both the **exposures and excretion abilities** for each of the two main forms of mercury we are exposed to. The QS Tri-Test utilizes mercury speciation analysis, a patented advanced technology that separates methyl mercury from inorganic mercury and measures each directly. This technique provides unprecedented information for the healthcare practitioner to assess the patient's difficulties with each form of mercury and plan a successful detoxification strategy.

The Analytical Suite and Results Reporting

The full analytical suite includes three tests: (1) mercury speciation analysis of patient's blood, (2) mercury speciation analysis of patient's urine, and (3) total mercury analysis of patient's hair.
Mercury speciation analysis shows 2 forms of mercury:

- Inorganic mercury (HgII) in blood usually reflects a dental amalgam exposure, though is also formed by the breakdown of methylmercury and its main excretion route is urine. The urine:blood ratio gives an index of excretion efficiency for inorganic mercury.
- Methylmercury (MeHg) reflects seafood consumption, though some is made in the gut from swallowed amalgam-based mercury. Excretion of methylmercury is reflected in the hair. The hair:blood ratio gives an index of excretion efficiency of methylmercury

Our customized reports contain raw and graphical data (sample, right). Each graphic provides references to help practitioners and patients interpret results.

Contact Information:

Quicksilver Scientific
1376 Miners Dr., Suite 101
Lafayette, CO 80026

Phone: 303-531-0861

Email: info@quicksilverscientific.com

Section V

Sang Whang and Alkalife

Sang Whang, inventor of Alkalife, is an engineer, scientist and inventor with many U.S. patents.

The Cancer Riddle
By Sang Whang

After billions of dollars and decades in time, we are not any closer to solving the cancer riddle, the number two killer in this country. Never mind solving or conquering cancer, we don't even understand the fundamental cause of cancer. WHY?

Is it possible that our whole approach to cancer is wrong? As a scientist who spent the past twenty years in the research of scientific reasons for human diseases, I say we are missing one essential element: ACID. It is the excess acid in our body that cultivates cancer. The scientific facts are: 1) cancer cells are acidic while healthy cells are alkaline, 2) an acidic environment contains less oxygen than an alkaline environment, 3) healthy cells die in an acidic environment while cancer cells die in an alkaline environment.

It is clear that research on cancer should start from changing an acidic environment to an alkaline environment and then to see the effects of environmental change on cancer cells. Why hasn't this been done? Maybe it is because the concept is too simple. Western medicine does not understand the pH influence in our body. We look for very complicated solutions, which receive huge government research funds. So far these solutions only lead to the development of expensive drugs and complicated machineries, which in turn lead to side effects, requiring more research and more drugs. Am I being cynical? You bet I am. I am frustrated to see life cut short by cancer while billions of our tax dollars are wasted.

It is a scientific fact that when we apply highly concentrated alkaline solution (pH >13) to a skin cancer spot, the skin cancer cells die. The spot hurts and leaves an ugly red burnt mark; but when the new skin grows back, there is no sign of cancer. An interesting thing to note is that the surrounding healthy cells do not die. A high pH alkaline solution does not kill healthy cells like radiation or chemotherapy does. I do not recommend laymen treating their own skin cancer this way, but I do recommend that professional dermatologists experiment with different pH solutions and come up with treatments for different kinds of skin cancer.

If doctors can measure the size and the pH of a tumor, they should be able to calculate the number of mole of hydroxyl ions (OH-) needed to destroy the tumor without killing any healthy cells surrounding it. Sounds like science fiction. But with a fraction of the money that is being spent, we can find a way to accomplish this.

Another interesting scientific fact that helps us understand the human body's natural survival technique is the ability of human cells to multiply (mitosis). We are told that the average human body has about 75 trillion cells. Cells live about 4 weeks and die after mitosis, and one cell becomes two; however, after 4 weeks, our body does not have 150 trillion cells, but still 75 trillion cells. This means only half of the cells multiply and the other half must disintegrate or die. If 37.5 trillion cells die in 4 weeks, how many cells die in one week, one day, one hour, one minute and one second? More than 10 million cells die per second!

The law of nature is such that strong and healthy cells multiply; damaged, injured, infected, contaminated, radiated and weak cells die. This is how we are designed by the Creator to maintain health in this world of radiation, contamination, bacteria/viruses, carcinogens in foods and drinks, cellular phones, etc.

To maintain health, a healthy body must be capable of dumping all the dead cells, natural and man-made. Dead cells are acidic and require alkaline minerals or bicarbonate to neutralize them and be dumped safely through urine. They are the cause of diseases when we cannot dump them. Our exhaust system, therefore, requires plenty of bicarbonate.

Bicarbonate is an alkaline buffer that neutralizes excess acid in the blood and maintains a healthy blood pH value. Medical science has discovered that as we age, we lose bicarbonate in the blood, noticeably so after the age of 45. This is the average age when we begin to show signs of diabetes, hypertension, high cholesterol, osteoporosis, arthritis, kidney stones, migraine, and even cancer. The decline of bicarbonate in our blood is the cause of physiological aging. If we could charge bicarbonate to the blood -- like a battery charger charging electrons to a battery -- we could help the human body maintain good health and live longer.

As long as we do not increase our body's alkalinity, we will never solve the cancer riddle. Diet and exercise are not enough to make a significant change; we need effective bicarbonate chargers.

Alkalife International has developed three different products that charge bicarbonate to the blood: Alkalife®, Bicarb-Balance™, and e-Cal®. These three products are patented or patent-pending.

Alkalife® is the original alkaline concentrate to make ordinary drinking water alkaline (pH about 10) by adding a few drops of it to a glass of non-carbonated drinking water. When alkaline water goes into the stomach, stomach pH increases, inducing the stomach to produce more hydrochloric acid. When the stomach produces hydrochloric acid, it also produces bicarbonate and interjects it into the bloodstream; thus increasing the blood's bicarbonate content. The ingredients of Alkalife® are diluted potassium hydroxide and sodium hydroxide.

Bicarb-Balance™ is a tablet with the proper ratio of potassium bicarbonate and sodium bicarbonate in a time-release compound with enteric coating. Enteric coating is used to protect bicarbonates from being destroyed by hydrochloric acid in the stomach; the time-release compound adds bicarbonates slowly to the blood. For people on heart medication or kidney dialysis who cannot/should not take additional potassium, we do not recommend Bicarb-Balance™ nor Alkalife®; we recommend e-Cal®.

e-Cal® is a calcium carbonate tablet in a time-release compound with enteric coating. When calcium carbonate is delivered to the bloodstream the carbonic acid in the blood reacts with the calcium carbonate, dissolves it and converts it to calcium bicarbonate, the form that the body needs. The calcium carbonate in e-Cal® is impurity-free.

Alkalife TEN is a premium spring water, bottled at the source, infused with the Alkalife pH booster formula. It comes is in BPA free bottles that have been tested for over 20 months to hold their pH at 10.0. The water is from natural springs that start at a very low total dissolved solid (TDS). The water has no fluoride and is very low in calcium content. Alkalife TEN is a therapeutic water that is best consumed on an empty stomach. Drink 4 half liters or 2 liters of Alkalife TEN daily.

Aqua ION Liquid Water pH Tester is designed to test the pH of your water. By measuring your water pH, you can make sure that you are getting high pH 10 alkaline water.

AlkaBest Water Ionizer is a water ionizer that takes tap water and filters it through proprietary Aquaspace water filtration and produces high pH low ORP mineral rich water. AlkaBest produces a therapeutic water that should be consumed preferably on an empty stomach. Drink 5-6 eight ounce glasses of ionized alkaline water daily. This ionizer was developed by Sang Whang along with Michael Pedersen who developed water filtration with NASA on the Space Shuttle.

Caution

Acid coagulates blood, while a more alkaline environment allows blood to flow more freely. Because of this, our products tend to act much like natural blood thinners, only without the side effects. There is, however, a potential danger of overly thin blood if you take our products in conjunction with a prescribed blood thinner. The blood would need to be monitored periodically, just to make sure this is not happening. Also, because of the amount of potassium that is used in kidney dialysis, we recommend for dialysis patients to not take Alkalife or Bicarb-Balance. E-Cal is safer for them.

Please visit our website to read testimonials and more Science and Health Series articles by Sang Whang.

Contact Information:

Mailing address: Alkalife International
8888 SW 129 Terrace
Miami, FL 33176
USA

Local (Within US):1-888-261-0870 International: 1-305-235-5120

Website: www.alkalife.com   Email: Info@alkalife.com

Herbs

If herbs are part of your protocol, my choice would be
Renee Ponder Herbs.

RENÉE PONDER

Master Herbalist

Renée Ponder, Master Herbalist, has built a successful
consulting practice that harmoniously integrates nutrition
and herbs. Renée began her herbal journey over 20 years
ago, after attending Post Graduate School in Berkeley,
participating in numerous herbal courses and studying with
some of the United States' most renowned Herbalists. She
continues to update her education with extensive seminar
and course work. She has developed over 25 herbal
formulations, teas and kits exclusively for Renee Ponder
Herbs, Inc. These trademarked formulas have been used in
nutritional protocols by Practitioners for ailments ranging
from cancer, colds, flu, allergies, arthritis, menopause,
prostate health, and PMS. Renée's expertise lies in herbs
for cleansing, detoxification and building the immune
system. Renée has made a mission of pursuing sources for
the finest quality fresh and organic herbs, which she uses in
her hand made formulations. They are distributed through
Renee Ponder Herbs, Inc., a flourishing California small
business, of which she is founding President (1981).
Despite many lucrative offers to mass produce, she has

never compromised the standards of her product and insists on the quality that results from hand manufacturing. She is respected nationally as a motivational speaker and as an advocate for the use of fresh and organic herbs. She has built a large Practitioner clientele and provides Private Label formulations of outstanding quality.

Contact Information:

Renée can be contacted at 1-800-684-3722

PO Box 70, Forest Knolls, CA 94933

Email: Renee@ReneePonderHerbs.com

Website: www.reneeponderherbs.com

Thermography
Breast Health & Whole Body Imaging

"Early Detection Saves Lives"
Meditherm® Safe Infrared Technology
FDA approved
NO pain- NO Compression- NO Radiation

What is DITI?

Digital Infrared Thermal Imaging (DITI) is a 15 minute non- invasive test of physiology. It is a valuable procedure for alerting your doctor to changes that may indicate early stage breast disease.

The benefit of DITI testing is that it offers the opportunity of earlier detection of breast disease than has been possible through breast self-examination, doctor examination or mammography alone.

DITI detects the subtle physiologic changes that accompany breast pathology, whether it is cancer, fibrocystic disease, an infection or a vascular disease. Your doctor can then plan accordingly and lay out a careful program to further diagnose and/or monitor you during and after any treatment.

Procedure

Non-invasive
No radiation
Painless
No contact with the body
FDA registered

This quick and easy test starts with your medical history being taken before you partially disrobe for the scanning to be performed. This first session provides your "thermal signature". A subsequent session 3-4 months later establishes a baseline if the patterns remain stable and unchanged.

All of your thermograms (breast images) are kept on record and once your stable thermal pattern has been established any changes can be detected during routine annual studies.

Who?

All women can benefit from DITI breasts screening. However, it is especially appropriate for younger women (30-50) whose denser breast tissue makes it more difficult for mammography to be effective. Also for women of all ages who, for some reasons, are unable to undergo routine mammography. This test can provide a 'clinical marker' to the doctor or mammographer that a specific area of the breast needs particularly close examination.

It takes years for a tumor to grow thus the earliest possible indication of abnormality is needed to allow for the earliest possible treatment and intervention. DITI's role in monitoring breasts health is to help in early detection and monitoring of abnormal physiology.

Your results are reported quickly by medical doctors who are board certified in thermology and include all color images taken during your test.

Current Early Detection Guidelines

One day there may be a single method for the early detection of breast cancer. Until then, using a combination of methods will increase your chances of detecting cancer in an early stage. These methods include:

Annual DITI screening for women of all ages.

Mammography, when considered appropriate for women who are aged 50 or older.

A regular breast examination by a health professional.

Monthly breast self-examination.

Personal awareness for changes in the breasts.

Readiness to discuss quickly any such changes with a doctor.

These guidelines should be considered along with your background and medical history.

Contact information:

Food for Thought Thermography

Susan Bischak, CCT & Dona Garofano, ND, CCT
123 Skyline Drive
Ringwood, NJ 07456
973-838-7211
&
Vista Natural Wellness Center

Susan Bischak, CCT & Sheryl Brian, CCT
191 Ramapo Valley Road
Oakland, NJ 07436
201-644-0840

Websites: www.naturalharmonyinfo.com,
www.meditherm.com/breasthealth

<u>Juicing</u>

Juicing may be a big part of your life going through this whole experience. Surely you have heard throughout your life to "eat your fruits and vegetables". A perfect way to consume these disease fighting foods is to juice. The process of juicing breaks open the cell walls to release the most nutrition from whole foods.

Vita-Mix

The **Vita-Mix** blender is amazing. It is so powerful. In 60 seconds you can have such a healthy whole food juice full of fiber.

For more information and to purchase a **Vita-Mix** contact: Website: www.vitamix.com

Champion Juicer

The **Champion Juicer** makes it easier to eat healthier, more flavorful foods. Champion Juicer is 3rd generation family owned.

Health professionals praise the nutritional benefits of adding fresh juice from greens, vegetables and fruits as part of a balanced diet. Champion Juicer's faster juicing process results in a richer, deeper colored juice with more flavor and nutrients.

For more information and to purchase a **Champion Juicer** contact:

Corporate Headquarters:
PLASTAKET MFG. CO., INC. / Champion Juicer
6220 E. Highway 12
Lodi CA, 95240
USA

Website: www.championjuicer.com

Tel: 866-935-8423 / 209-369-2154

To find USA local farming in your area go to:
www.localharvest.org

If purchasing produce from a supermarket, take note to the stickers on the individual vegetable/fruit. The 1st # tells you how the produce was grown. Although these codes are used globally it is a voluntary system.

4 digit codes starting with #4 or #3 are conventionally grown by using pesticides.

5 digit codes starting with #9 are organically grown.

5 digit codes starting with #8 are Genetically Modified (GMO, GE).

*The preferable choice would be organic.

Sweating

The way the body releases toxins physically is through perspiration, respiration, defecation and urination. Some of the entities included in The Gift of *Options* for the most part will address these areas.

Depending upon your state of health and energy level, it may be difficult for you to perform any kind of exercise. It is still important for you to sweat. An infrared sauna will help sweat those toxins out by just sitting. There are infrared saunas available for home use. However, this may not be accessible in your home. Contact health spas, chiropractors, naturopaths and yoga centers to see if they have infrared saunas and can purchase sessions from them. Sipping on water with electrolytes in a glass or stainless steel container while you are in a sauna may be helpful (notice that plastic was not included). As your body is sweating and releasing toxins, you need to replenish your fluids with nutrients. Don't drink anything with artificial anything. It is recommended that you seek clearance from your doctor or licensed practitioner before use.

I welcome your feedback about your progress and any suggestions you may have. Please correspond through email.

Contact Information:

Email: thegiftofoptions@gmail.com

Follow me on my Blog:
http://thegiftofoptions.blogspot.com

I Leave You With This Final Note:

Dare to step outside of your comfort zone. Reach deep inside where there lies infinite possibilities available to everyone.

Enjoy the ride, keep smiling and love!

~Toni Kimble

About the Author

The process of researching health-related issues is very familiar to Toni. As a person who never felt well growing up, she searched for years to improve her health. While she had no serious illnesses, she was faced on a daily basis with annoying symptoms that held her back from a daily routine to which any average healthy person wouldn't give a second thought. Her wish is that this resource, The Gift of *Options* helps many.